CLEAN EATING
GUIDE

A Simple Way to Achieve Healthy Weight Loss

(Healthy and Delicious Recipe Tips for Eating Clean)

Robert Harmon

Published by Alex Howard

Clean Eating Guide: A Simple Way to Achieve Healthy Weight Loss
(Healthy and Delicious Recipe Tips for Eating Clean)

ISBN 978-1-990169-04-5

Legal & Disclaimer

The information contained in this book is not designed to replace or take the place of any form of medicine or professional medical advice. The information in this book has been provided for educational and entertainment purposes only.

Table of contents

Part 1

Introduction

In "Clean Eating Guide" you will find a step by step approach that will help you to break your current eating habits and patterns and learn to "eat clean" to lose weight, improve your mood and, most importantly, prevent disease.

You are reading a crash course on clean eating and the minimalist lifestyle. This book explores several aspects of a healthy natural diet that average people struggle with.

I've included tips on clean diet preparation and food shopping, ways to meet your healthy eating goals on a day-to-day basis, morning-to-evening recipes, and methodologies for minimalist and mindful living. I've written it not from the perspective of someone who hasn't been in your shoes, but from that of an overweight person who grew up with an unhealthy relationship with food.

Combined with tons of love, "Clean Eating Guide" will help you reset your health, detox your body and empower you to make easy-to-prepare meals that your entire family will love.

My goal in writing this book is to start a conversation about the Clean Eating lifestyle. It's not meant to be something for you and a handful of other people only to think about; ideally, it's also a way to end an epidemic of eating disorders that are spreading around the world. Instead of applying clean-eating as part of a short-term diet, I'd rather see it become a complete solution to end irrational eating.

Today, the whole world is dealing with a dietary crisis caused by sugar and toxic substances: our food is laden with harmful ingredients designed to trigger harmful addictions and emotional eating. The obvious result is today's overwhelming increase in obesity.

If we observe our nation's relationship with food, we will find that fat is not the problem, and excess weight is not the end result. We need to find a genuinely clean approach, one that incorporates the consumption of nourishing and nutrition-rich foods as opposed to the hollow and empty foods that are so readily available in the market.

This practice of eating clean foods (foods that are closest to their natural state) has been embraced by celebrities, athletes and bodybuilders, but is still relatively new to the general public. "Clean Eating Guide" will teach you to pick up a piece of fruit instead of a fruit-flavored something for a snack. It will help you say goodbye to empty carbs and sugar- and additive-laden foods.

If you ask me to describe Clean Eating, I'll use two words: awareness and mindfulness. "Acceptance with awareness of your body and whole life each and every moment, by mindfully living in the present and savoring the gifts the present moment offers." Using this principle, you will expand your knowledge about the clean lifestyle. That's the main reason why this book also focuses on meditation and deep breathing.

I'm delighted that you've chosen to read this book. It may be the first step you take to empower yourself to meet your goals of being healthier and happier.

If I can do it, so can you!

Chapter 1: Resetting Your System

How Clean Eating Does Your Body A World Of Good

I am so glad you are reading this book. Whatever is your reason for doing so -maybe you wish to wipe the slate clean, detox your system, lose a ton of weight, or simply boost your energy levels- you have taken the first step in the right direction.

I have kept things simple, so this book is for everyone who wishes to hit 'reset' on their junk-filled systems. I will briefly share my story and experiences with traditional diets and how clean and holistic eating along with minimalism turned out to be the most realistic approach that not only worked for me; it changed my entire family's approach towards eating.

"How do you stay so skinny?"

"You must have an amazing metabolism!"

I wish I could tell every person who says those things to me how further from the truth they are. I was not one of those lucky people who have a high metabolism which allows them to tuck in whatever they like without gaining an ounce of fat on their body. By the time I was 35, following the birth of my second son, I had gained a whopping 40 pounds over and above the average weight for my BMI.

Then began a long and difficult journey to lose all that extra weight. Like most people, I tried a variety of diets and weight loss workouts. In the beginning, I did see results. But the trouble always lay in keeping the weight off. Whatever your personal weight loss story may be, I am sure you identify with what I went through each time a diet failed.

Now, I am not a doctor, a chef or a dietician. I am an average, 40-year-old working mother of two kids. Like most of you, I turned to food when a diet failed. I was no longer looking at food as a means of keeping me alive, but for emotional and social security.

In 2014, I happened to sign up for a meditation course where it was mandatory that attendees avoid meat, eggs, caffeine and alcohol for the entire duration of the course. I did so meticulously.

By the time the course ended, I had realized that my relationship with myself had changed. I was more loving, more compassionate and more confident in my dealings with others as well as the way I viewed myself. It might have been the result of the processes we underwent during the course, or it could be the spiritual discourses on the importance of living minimally held at the end of each day of the course- one thing became clearer to me: my food and lifestyle were affecting me in unimaginable ways. They most definitely were affecting my Prana or life energy.

Those 10 days helped me realize that- all through the course when I had lain off junk and non-vegetarian food, I felt a lot more energetic; I slept better, my headaches and food cravings were gone. I felt happier. I felt lighter. I was in love- with myself!

We, course attendees, were also asked to practice the meditation techniques and food habits we had picked up during the course for a period of at least 40 days. It is said that when you do something for 40 days, you have a better chance of sticking with it for life.

At the end of the 40th day, I had made a decision that changed my life. I decided to give up all the animal-based and processed foods that I was so used to eat. I decided to adopt clean and holistic eating practices into my life. As my meditation practice grew daily, I started shopping smarter, preparing food more holistically and encouraged my family also to adopt these changes.

We started learning about minimalism, thinking carefully before making mindless purchases. I am glad that my husband also took up the same meditation course. He too has discovered the happiness, and lightness meditation brings. Since my children were young then, changing their eating habits was not very difficult to do. As a result, our entire family turned to clean eating and holistic living.

Over the past years, (it has been two beautiful years since I participated in the course) I lost a lot of weight and today, I receive many compliments for the way I look. People who didn't see me in a while come up to me and tell me how younger I look and "there is a certain light in my eyes!"

Today, when I look back, I realize what an unhealthy relationship I had with food. It has helped us rethink our choices not to mention the way my family has started approaching all decisions.

The clean lifestyle is not just about eating; it is about holistic practices that do not harm nature or the environment around us. It is about making choices that do not involve harming animals. You might say, "How can one or two families living clean change the world!" The fact is: clean eating and the holistic tribe are increasing. I am so glad to see more and more people realizing the amazing health benefits of such a clean lifestyle.

Make no mistake: this book isn't about veganism or vegetarianism, but my readers would be glad to note that the recipes discussed herein do conform to the vegetarian and vegan lifestyle.

Over the years, I have learned to address nutrition from all angles. Today, my family reads food labels meticulously focusing on wholesome, unprocessed foods.

In fact, we live by five simple rules:

1.Pick foods that are closest to nature as possible

The more processed stuff you put into your mouth; the greater is the likelihood of consuming harmful ingredients that are straight out of the lab.

2.Eat a rainbow colored platter of fruits and veggies

The more colors you have on your plate, the better.

3.Choose local and seasonal products

There is a reason why certain foods grow only in certain areas and certain seasons. They provide the nutrients your body needs and actually taste a lot better when eaten in season.

4.Choose companies that adopt green practices

Learn all you can about the companies you source your food from. It does pay to visit their websites and read media reports about them.

5.Eat together-eat with gratitude

Savor every morsel of food that you eat. Prepare the food with love. After all; only correctly prepared food can nourish your body and mind. Savoring the food's flavor and taste will also help you eat mindfully instead of eating to satisfy cravings.

Benefits Of Clean Eating

A great deal has been said about clean eating-eating foods closest to their natural states. Eating clean organic, wholesome foods can help you fight diseases, lose weight, live longer and also become happier. These promises might sound like those coming straight out of an afternoon infomercial but they are all true nevertheless, and I vouch for them.

Here are benefits of clean eating in a nutshell:

1.Good health and immunity

If you have been blessed with good health, then you are indeed blessed! Not all of us are lucky in that way. I had battled migraines and PMS before I adopted a clean, minimalist lifestyle. Yes, genes do play an important role in many diseases, but a large part of those diseases can be prevented by controlling one's diet. Diet has a significant role in disease prevention. For example, the majority of cancers are now known to be caused by eating red meat. Also, eating sugar, unhealthy fats, and alcohol have been linked to decreased efficiency of the immune system.

2.Prevention of obesity

Plant-based diets like vegan and vegetarian diets are considered as world's best diets for the simple reason: they really help you lose weight. A study was conducted on different diets to determine their efficacy in losing weight. The results clearly showed that plant-based diets such as Veganism proved much more effective than other low calorie or elimination diets that allowed animal products.

3.Diabetes prevention

Vegetarians and vegans have approximately half the risk of developing diabetes. A study indicated that vegans only had 2.9% prevalence of developing diabetes as compared to 7.6% in non-vegetarians.

4.Prevention of heart disease

In clinical trials, plant-based clean diets showed regression in atherosclerosis or hardening of arteries.

5.Reduced Cravings

Sugar is addictive- the more you eat it, the more you want it. Just three weeks of clean eating has been known to get people off sugar cravings for good.

6.Hair, skin health and anti-aging benefits

Since you eat a wide range of healthy and fresh fruits and vegetables, you start noticing an improvement in your hair, skin and nails. Anti-aging benefits are also inevitable since you reduce toxins and free radicals that age you prematurely.

7.Reduced ADD and ADHD

It is no secret that ADD and ADHD are both caused by preservatives, dyes, sugar and gluten rich foods. Many patients suffering from Attention Deficit Disorders have reduced temper tantrums and mood swings by eating clean.

The clean eating plan can thus help you stay mentally alert and improve memory and concentration. Its focus is on eating a variety of clean, wholesome foods that pack a nutritious punch.

No matter what your current state of health is: you will see a world of difference in your life by adopting the clean eating lifestyle. You can normalize your weight, blood pressure readings and also reduce your overall cholesterol. You will have improved digestion, clearer skin, and mental sharpness.

Even if you are already blessed with good health, you can clean eat your way to maintain your health. Yes, I promise that you will tip the balance in your favor by eating and living in this manner.

In the next chapter, we will look at what clean eating is all about.

Chapter 2: What Is Clean Eating All About?

I am going to be very honest with you. The clean and minimalist lifestyle is not easy. It means that you, or whoever you live with, will be cooking- quite a lot. However, you mustn't let this fact deter you. A weekly outline plan will help you come up with the right meals and, with some practice; you can adjust to this lifestyle very easily. The most important thing is that you will start experiencing so many benefits that you will feel encouraged to adapt very easily to this change.

In this chapter, I will highlight all the basics of clean eating which will help you stick to this path. Remember: the clean eating minimalist lifestyle is ever-evolving and, like us, it is a work in progress. Here, we will briefly cover the basic principles of eating clean, why we should say No to certain food groups and also briefly touch base on some points to help you take baby steps in the right direction.

Some points to note before we proceed:

•This book is not a resource for crash dieting

•This lifestyle that I am chalking out for you will help you come up with your own sustainable, healthy eating plan.

Whatever I have discussed here is what I practice myself. Finding fun and healthy ways to incorporate clean meals in daily life has become a part of my life as it will become yours. I hope you have as much fun as I do in doing so. So do not complain that it is time-consuming – it may be, but it is the most important thing you will do for healthy mind and body.

When I talk about clean living, here is what I mean:

• Eating healthy, balanced, usually self-prepared meals

• Lots of fruits and vegetables

• Healthy fats and vegetarian protein in every meal

• Eating a wide range of plant-based foods

• Including healthy low Glycemic Index carbs. Low GI foods are complex carbohydrates which, unlike simple carbs, do not spike up your blood sugar levels. Rather, they deliver slow release of energy, so you feel full longer, and you do not experience food cravings.

• Not pressurizing you or your family members to take up the lifestyle. There will be days when you slip- the key is to get back on track instead of beating yourself against the wall. You will notice that the cleaner you eat, the fewer your cravings will be. The more your body gets real nutrition, the less it will desire the unhealthy foods that lead to greater cravings.

•Reducing toxic overload by selecting organic household cleaners etc..

•Meditation and mindfulness- I cannot stress how important this is in practicing the clean and healthy lifestyle. The mind plays an important role in the body's well being. The cleaner your thoughts, the better your choices will be in all aspects and not just the diet.

What Does Clean Eating Mean?

Eating clean does not mean cleaning your food before you eat it. As most of you probably already know, clean eating means selecting foods that are as close as possible to their natural state. It means eating whole foods such as fruits and vegetables, nuts and seeds, legumes and whole grains.

Why give up meat and non-vegetarian foods?

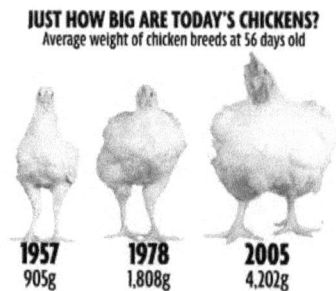

JUST HOW BIG ARE TODAY'S CHICKENS?
Average weight of chicken breeds at 56 days old

1957	1978	2005
905g	1,808g	4,202g

We cannot eat meat raw. The meat consumed today is filled with tons of hormones. If you visit chicken farms, you will be shocked to see the conditions under which the poultry is bred.

Do you know what the animals and birds go through when they are taken to the slaughterhouse? Don't you think that all that negativity actually manifests into their body and unknowingly passes into the food as well?

Did you also know that gallons of water go into the processing of your hamburgers? Do you realize the amount of damage your food choices are inflicting upon the earth and Mother Nature?

Do you remember the big earthquake of Nepal? What does that have to do with the topic at hand? You will be shocked to find out that there is a link. Every year, Nepal hosts an animal butchering Gadhimai festival where millions of birds and animals are slaughtered for food and appeasing the Gods. Seismographs actually show that the shrieks and cries of animals being butchered actually go and hit the tectonic plates in the area causing massive amounts of pressure to build up in them.

This is actually based on Einstein's Pain Wave Theory. The pressure reaches a tipping point causing earthquakes, tsunamis, and other calamities. Thousands of lives were lost in Nepal's earthquake not to mention the massive damage to property. I would not want to say that Nepal brought this tragedy upon herself. I am indeed very sorry for all that destruction of life and property, but I feel there will come a time when Mother Nature will heed the cries of her weaker children.

Man Is Not Meant To Be A Meat Eater

If you study the diet of the prehistoric men and women, it can be seen that their primary diet was meat. The Paleolithic era man never survived beyond the average lifespan of 30 years. This really makes me question the logic behind the popular Paleo and Ketogenic diets which primarily focus on meat and animal proteins.

I do not want to get into a debate about diets. The main reason why I am bringing this up is to point out the fact that our intestines are just not made for consuming animal foods like meat, milk, eggs, etc.

The Creator made man, He did so with complete vegetarianism in mind. Our intestines are much larger compared to the carnivores' intestines. This is because, they are not designed to handle meat; rather they are meant to eat grains, legumes, fruits and vegetables which are easily digested and passed off quickly. Animal-based foods take much longer to digest: almost 72 hours.

This is the main reason why the intestines in carnivores are a lot smaller compared to those in herbivores in order to help them pass out the heavy food. This is also the reason why Thanksgiving meals make us feel bloated, heavy, and drowsy. So the first rule of cleaner eating is eliminating meat from the diet.

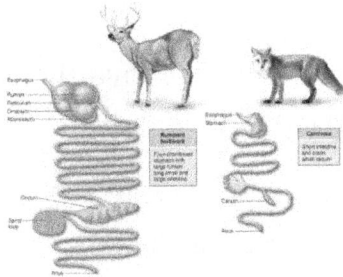

The Truth About Dairy

Man is the only animal that drinks milk belonging to another animal. Just think about it- how unnatural that is! Today we are drinking cow, buffalo, camel, and even goat's milk. Tomorrow, we might as well consider milking our pet cat or dog! Gross! Why then would you find it natural to drink the milk of a cow? How different is that from drinking your cat's milk?

Did you know that the majority of hormonal imbalances that people suffer from today are attributed to their consumption of dairy products? Dairy is known to cause acne breakouts in teenagers, and even adults are breaking out in their 30s and 40s!

Dairy and dairy products are full of hormones that are meant to be passed from the mother cow to her newborn calf for its growth and development. Imagine you are drinking milk filled with all those hormones!

That is the main reason why, when we started the clean eating lifestyle we first cut dairy and meat from our lives. Think of clean eating and minimalism as de-clutter of sorts: you must remove the clutter from your kitchen, pantry, from your lives and from your mind.

It is very simple: people reach out for the first thing they see when they are hungry. If your pantry is stocked with clean, wholesome foods, then that is what you will reach out for. I know it sounds tough, but it is all about practice. I cannot reiterate that enough.

Here are some top tips to help you reinforce these principles:

•Eat foods made by nature- if it is manmade-toss it out

•Avoid everything that comes in a packet or a box

•Use healthy cooking means

•Eat before you get hungry

•Do not measure your portions or watch your calories

•Eat slowly and mindfully- listen to your brain. If you are full, stop eating.

Whole Versus Processed: The Science

Artificial colors

Xylitol

Sodium alginate

Artificial flavor

Milk protein concentrate

These are actual ingredients listed in a popular sugar-free pudding. Why would you want to eat such a pudding which has ingredients that one cannot even pronounce? Manufacturers strip off many foods to make them more edible and also have longer shelf life.

Conversely, clean whole foods come in their natural form with tons of flavor, color, and nutrients. Manufacturers add texture and flavors to enhance the taste of foods. These factors, along with tons of added sugar and salt, make processed foods highly addictive in nature. These artificial processes used during food manufacturing make them so pleasing to the palate that you simply cannot stop eating them. This leads to binge eating and obesity.

The foods I want you to start stocking up from today are the ones that are minimally processed. They won't come with an ingredient list- neither will they come with preparation instructions.

Naturally, there will be times when you will come across certain minimally processed foods such as whole grain pasta, but processed nonetheless. Do get into a habit of reading food labels. I will subsequently help you out with many tips to help you stock a clean eating kitchen- these tips will definitely prepare you for your trip to the grocery store.

Starting Out: Taking Baby Steps

As I have stated before, transitioning to the clean eating lifestyle is not an easy task. It will certainly not happen overnight. I will encourage you to start in very small steps as below:

•Step 1: Start with one clean meal per week. This will help you wean reluctant family members.

•Step 2: Add another clean meal.

•Step 3: Out of 7 dinners which the entire family eats together, try and get to 50% i.e. at least 4 meals that are clean. Make your potato chips at home instead of getting them out of a bag.

•Step 4: You and your family are convinced this is the lifestyle for you. So completely toss out the garbage and stop buying processed stuff. You will be amazed at the money you are saving as you stop eating out.

•Step 5: You are at 80-90% clean. The majority of your meals are made at home not to count the bottle of pasta sauce and store-bought bread.

•Step 6: You go 100% clean. This is the option for people who are sick and tired of being so. Most people at this stage still eat out once in a while.

All this might seem a bit difficult and like I have stated many times before that the process will take time. Be patient. There is no way out of the processed food maze but with the right thought and efforts, you can help get your family on the clean eating bandwagon too.

One of the best parts of this lifestyle is that you will feel so much healthier and happier that you will go on an upward spiral of well-being rather than being pulled into a downward spiral of disease and depression.

Chapter 3: Preparing For The Clean Diet

This is where we get down to the nitty-gritty of the clean lifestyle.

There is an old adage that goes: "Teach a man to fish and you will feed him for a lifetime". From my experience of transitioning to the clean living and minimalism lifestyle, I know that the first few weeks can make all the difference. In this case, it could be the difference between looking good and feeling great in those weeks to making a reach change that positively reverberates affecting everyone it touches.

It is always a good idea to note down your progress. There are a couple of ways to do so. I like to keep a food journal and a diary where I note down days that I ate clean completely. You can also print out a calendar and keep it on the refrigerator. Mark a star on the days you ate clean and a cross on the days you had even one processed item. Or you can use the ready shopping item lists below to print out and take to the store.

Remember: clean eaters always shop around the perimeter of the grocery stores- that is where the best and most natural items are stocked.

Best Places To Shop For Clean Ingredients

- Whole Foods

- Trader Joe's

- Sprouts

- Mothers

- Amazon

- Safeway

You must also invest in some basic clean eating tools like blenders, food processor, dehydrator, etc. Also, buy a slow cooker if you do not have one. This will keep your meals warm, and you need not stand over the meal waiting for it to get ready. I have not included any slow cooker recipes here, but I certainly have a collection ready for another e-book.

Must Have Shopping Items For Your Clean Eating Pantry (Print This List Out)

1.Always shop the perimeter of your store. This is where the nutritious foods are at!

2.Read labels- go for non GMO (genetically modified) whole products. Avoid franken-soy or soy products made from Monsanto's RoundUp soyabean.

3.Support local farmers and traders as far as possible.

Vegetables, leafy greens, sprouts, herbs and tubers

•Artichokes

•Arugula

•Asparagus

•Beets

•Broccoli

•Bok Choy

•Carrots

•Cilantro

•Collard greens

•Chives

•Cauliflower

•Cabbage

•Celery

•Cucumbers

- Chard

- Bell peppers

- Brussels Sprouts

- Eggplant

- Garlic

- Ginger

- Green beans

- Green peas

- Green onions

- Jalapenos

- Kale

- Lavender

- Lettuce greens

- Mushrooms

- Mustard greens

- Okra

- Oregano

- Parsnips

- Parsley

- Potatoes

- Pumpkins

- Red Onions

- Radish

- Rosemary

- Rutabaga

- Snap peas

- Squash

- Sweet Potatoes

- Shallots

- Spinach

- Turnips

- Thyme

- Yams

- Yucca roots

- White onions

- Zucchini

Sea vegetables (buy from Maine Seaweed Company, Eden Foods, Emerald Cove Sea Gift's Roasted Seaweed Snacks)

- Agar

- Arame

- Dulse

- Hiziki

- Kombu

- Nori

- Wakame

Fruits

- Apples

- Apricots

- Avocados

- Bananas

- Blueberries

- Blackberries

- Cantaloupes

- Cherries

- Citrus fruits

- Cranberries

- Currants

- Coconut

- Dragon fruit

- Figs

- Grapes

- Grapefruits

- Goji berries (add them to your smoothies)

- Kiwi fruit

- Lemons

- Limes

- Melons

- Mangos

- Mandarin

- Nectarines

- Oranges

- Passion fruit

- Pears

- Peaches

- Pineapples

- Plums

- Pomegranates

- Persimmon

- Raspberries

- Strawberries

- Tomatoes (plum, cherries and grape tomatoes)

- Watermelon

- Watercress

Nuts and seeds

- Almonds

- Brazil nuts

- Cashew nuts

- Chestnuts

- Chia seeds (makes a great smoothie)

- Flaxseeds

- Hazelnuts

- Hemp seeds

- Macadamia nuts

- Peanuts

- Pine nuts

- Pecans

- Pistachios

- Poppy seeds

- Pumpkin seeds

- Sunflower seeds

- Walnuts

Beans and legumes

- Adzuki beans

- Anasazi beans

- Black beans

- Black-eyed beans

- Cranberry beans

- Cannellini beans

- Chick peas

- Edamame (non GMO)

- Fava beans

- Garbanzo beans

- Kidney beans

- Lentils

- Lima beans

- Mothbeans

- Mung beans

- Navy beans

- Pinto beans

- Red beans

- Split peas

- White peas

- Yellow peas

Whole grains

•Brown rice

•Gluten free couscous

•Quinoa

•Rolled oats

•Steel cut oats

•Wheat berries

•Wild rice

Fats

•Coconut oil

•Olive oil

•Ghee

•Avocado oil

•Almond butter

•Extra virgin olive oil

•Salad dressing oils like walnut oil, hazel nut oils etc

Non dairy milk

- Soy milk

- Almond milk

- Flax milk

Flours, powders and breads

- Whole wheat flour

- Whole wheat pastry flour for muffins and baking

- Chickpea flour (this is gluten free and readily available at Indian or Pakistani stores)

- Buckwheat

- Sorghum

- Millet

- Amaranth flour

- Almond meal and almond flour

- Coconut flour (This is great for baking)

- Seitan (This is a great substitute for meat. It is the Japanese gluten obtained after washing starch and bran from whole wheat flour. It is available in natural food stores. It is very versatile and can be chopped, cubed, cut into strips for adding to soups, stews etc., as well as for stuffing as meat).

- Teff

- Kamut

- Ezekiel bread and tortilla (I recommend this to newbies to clean eating until you start baking your bread)

- Pita bread (from Trader Joe's)

- Acai powder

- Spirulina powder (this is a great source of protein)

- Carob powder

- Hemp powder

Beverages

- Water

- Herbal tea

- Decaffeinated tea and coffee

- Matcha and green tea (check caffeine content)

- Kefir

- Kombucha

- Coconut water

- Unsweetened coconut milk/almond milk

Necessities to have on hand always (sweeteners, spice and all things nice!)

•Coconut cream

•Coconut flakes

•Cinnamon

•Cayenne

•Raw cacao nibs and cocoa/cacao powder (unsweetened, organic)

•Maca powder (great to add to smoothies)

•Stevia and stevia leaves

•Agave nectar

•Turmeric

•Curry powder

•Organic vegetable broth (you can make this at home)

•Organic raw Apple Cider Vinegar

•Organic pure, raw Maple syrup

•Maple sugar

•Balsamic Vinegar

•Tamari to use in place of Soy sauce

•Pink Himalayan salt or sea salt or rock salt

•Dijon Mustard

•Mejdool dates

•Fresh and dried fruits

•Coconut palm sugar

•Miso

•Soy sauce (choose reduced sodium, high quality soy sauce) or you can cook with fermented Tamari and Shoyu sauces. These are readily available in natural food stores).

•Pure Vanilla extract

Plant based, clean ready to eat snacks

•Ezekiel bread and Ezekiel tortillas (I do not eat these, but I recommend these to people new to clean eating. They do contain gluten but these are healthier alternatives to other commercial breads. They are made with sprouted grains and are great for people missing their breads).

•Hummus

•Daiya dairy free pepper jack shreds

•Raw chocolate (Gnosis or Nibmor)

•Pretzels (We love Mary's Gone Crackers Sticks and Twigs)

•Amy's frozen burritos

For kids

•Frozen fruit smoothies

•Ak Mak whole wheat crackers (Note that these are not gluten free)

•Organic tomato sauce and pizza/pasta sauce (Eden Organic)

•Bagged frozen vegetables

•Amy's organic soups

•Gluten-free pizza crust (Udi's)

•Enjoy Life Cookies

•Organic peanut butter.

Note: If you are a meat lover who is transitioning to the vegan/vegetarian lifestyle, I recommend starting slowly. Add some lean proteins to your meals such as organic, cruelty-free eggs. However, it is important that you stay away from pre-packaged meats. You may choose organic, grass fed and cage free chicken or turkey where needed. You also can eat some soft cheeses but go for the low-fat ones. Keep your sugar intake minimal and watch out for products containing high fructose corn syrup.

Foods to stay away from

1.All artificial substances including artificial colors, flavors, and preservatives

2.All artificial sweeteners

3.All sugary drinks like pop, sodas, and diet beverages

4.Trans fats and fat substitutes

5.All items labeled low fat and low calorie- Manufacturers add many other ingredients to such foods to make up for the taste and flavor of fats

6.All non-fat items- These use processed artificial substances such as additives and starches to mimic flavor and texture of fats

Cooking Tips

•The main thing about clean eating is to eat everything raw-including broccoli.

•You can start small. Make a green smoothie with raw fruits and veggies in the morning. I like to roast everything we eat.

•Steaming, baking, and grilling are great options too. Steaming does take away nutrition, but a little bit of it is great if that can help you get your veggies down. The key to steaming is to do it very lightly. You do not want to over-steam veggies into a mushy paste.

•Baking is easy and fun too, and you can involve kids in it. Toss all your veggies with a bit of olive oil into the over and you have agreat side dish or snack.

•You will be eating a lot of beans and chickpeas, and I have many recipes included of them. You can use canned beans and chickpeas, but it is best that you soak them weekly and cook them ahead. This way, you can readily use them salads, soups, stews, etc.

The main, rather revolutionary idea behind clean eating is to cook your meals at home. In the later chapters, we will be dealing with some essential recipes which can help you cook in bulk. I know that this might seem time-consuming, but there are strategic ways for planning things.

41

To make life easier here are some top tips:

- Prep in advance so as to save a lot of time- I cook a little throughout the week and mostly on weekends instead of doing everything on one day. I add a lot of fresh or frozen veggies to meals as I go.

- I have included many snack recipes- Vegetable chips can be made without oil in a dehydrator in large batches. I suggest you invest in one.

- Pre-bagged organic fruit- Add them to smoothies or eat them as is.

- Green smoothies- I have discussed some recipes that are great for breakfast, lunch and dinner. Those who eat yogurt and other dairy products can also make milkshakes and whey protein shakes. I follow a plant based diet only so; I avoid these ingredients.

- Pre-cut carrots and celery sticks- These are great to snack on, and you can add them to your soups and stews or kids' meals and lunch boxes. Serve them with homemade Tahini and hummus.

- Homemade vegan protein bars- They are great for days you have no time for breakfast. I have discussed a no-bake protein bar recipe in the Recipes chapter.

- Avocado- It is packed with so much of good stuff- antioxidants, healthy fats, and fiber and so on. Make a large batch of guacamole and keep in the refrigerator.

•Mixed green salads- Buy a large bag of these and keep them handy as a quick side dish to bean soups, etc..

•A big batch of oatmeal- Make it ahead so you have four to five servings for the morning rush. Snack or breakfast on it by adding fresh berries.

Weekly Outline

•Pick simple recipes. Double the recipes so you can stock them in the refrigerator.

•Plan your complete week. As I said at the beginning of the chapter, note your progress. Sit with a calendar. Fill in one day with a circle on which you can cook ahead for the rest of the week. This way, you will have enough time for other things, especially if you have a busy day on which you are too tired to cook.

•Always buy items you can use in several recipes such as green smoothies.

•Make a shopping list based on the items given above. Tick off the things you need. Buy those items in bulk that last longer. Things such as greens do not last for more than three days so prepare them before they spoil. You can even make vegetable stock and keep.

•Make sure everyone in the family eats breakfast. It is the most important meal of the day. I will discuss some important clean breakfast recipes soon. Sprouted grain bread and overnight oatmeal are excellent choices. The soaking and sprouting make it easier to digest the meal.

•Always include a side dish of quinoa, sweet potatoes brown rice and other healthy carbs in main meals. Fill your plate with 50% slow burning, low GI vegetables

(More about GI or Glycemic Index in the following chapter).

•Seaweed- Seaweed is an essential source of minerals like iodine, calcium, and iron. It decreases the acidity of the body and boosts metabolism. It is a must have on your plate if you are looking to lose weight.

•Aim to get 30-50% fiber daily.

•Have a variety of nuts. Nuts are amazing, and you can simply eat them roasted or as is. Avoid salty nuts, though. You can also roast nuts and process them into creamy, nutty sauces and yogurt replacement.

•Keep healthy snacks on hand. Snacks do not mean those over-hyped health bars that contain tons of preservatives. Be mindful of the sugar content of these items. Sugar and chemicals are snuck into these foods. I will discuss homemade plant-based snack recipes shortly.

•Those who are not vegan may enjoy yogurt. Go for non-sugary and non-flavored yogurt.

•Homemade protein bars, protein shakes, fruits, dried fruits, green smoothies are ideal for snacking upon. They keep you full longer and are packed with tons of good stuff.

•Eat three meals and two snacks every day (adults). Keep total calorie intake for the day between 1,500-1,700 calories.

•Drink tons of water every day. Encourage your kids to do so as well. If they do not like plain water, fresh fruit juices are your best options.

•You should ideally meditate every day. We will be covering meditation and mindfulness and the role they play in later chapters.

Eating Out Tips

•Ask for sauces to be served on the side.

•Call the restaurant ahead asking if they can prepare meals in a clean manner with minimal processing. Remember: you have every right as a customer to ask for what you want.

•Ask for broiled, steamed or grilled foods.

•Many Chinese, Thai and Indian foods offer delicious plant-based meals made with tofu, beans, chickpeas, tempeh, etc. If you are vegan, avoid ghee (clarified butter used in Indian dishes) and yogurt.

•Ask for extra vegetables on the side instead of bread, pasta, etc.

•When eating at a friend's place: it is best to have small servings of everything served rather than denying or feeling deprived.

•Be polite, yet assertive in declining foods.

•Set an example- offer to bring a healthy dish along.

In the next chapter, we will discuss how to get the most out of the clean eating diet.

Chapter 4: Tips For Getting The Most Out Of The Clean Eating Diet

Over the last two years on the clean living lifestyle, we have learned many important lessons:

Food talks to our genes. It controls gene expression, metabolism, and hormones. What we eat has the potential to make us sick and gain weight. Eating an artificial processed food item like a cookie versus eating a handful of raw almonds can actually turn on disease-causing genes.

Over the past few years, I have interacted with many prominent members of the clean eating, plant-based diet community. Some of the more advanced ones have even omitted whole grains from their diet. I leave it entirely up to you to decide if you plan on including/not including grains.

The key is to focus on the glycemic index. (For those of you unaware of glycemic index or GI- it is the food's ability to cause a sugar spike in the blood. I believe this is the key factor in weight loss and obesity as well as other lifestyle diseases including diabetes.) Understanding GI overload is as important, if not more, as counting calories. My nutritionally balanced recipes below are complete balanced meals, and they have low glycemic overload.

What About Protein?

When I mentioned to my extended family that we planned to give up animal proteins completely, many scoffed at the idea. The question foremost on their mind was: "How the heck do you plan to give protein to the kids?"

There are many vegan and vegetarian sources of proteins. Many of them are, in fact, being considered as the best proteins to lose weight. I suggest you stock up on non-GMO (Genetically modified organisms) soy, tempeh, and tofu. Include at least two to three servings of soy protein daily in your diet. Stay away from artificial soy patties, burgers, and meatless chicken. They are packed with preservatives and artificial flavors.

There are also many supplements without Whey available in the market. These include pea and brown rice protein powders, and they are delicious. Do watch out for artificial flavors, though!

Eat nuts as well since they are packed with proteins and good fats. Chia seeds, sunflower and pumpkin seeds, almonds, pistachios, and walnuts are excellent sources of proteins and omega 3.

Start sprouting. Not a day goes by when we do not sprout something or the other. Sprouting beans, seeds, and grains increase their nutritional value multifold.

Know Your Food Combining Secrets

There is a science behind food combination. Combining food groups helps your system digest food better. It also helps the body absorb nutrients and complements each other to enhance their nutritional values.

Here are a few food combining rules:

•Combine carbohydrate with fiber.

•Combine protein with anti-inflammatory fats like coconut oil, olive oil, and avocado.

Calcium

The good news is that you do not need to depend on milk and milk products to get your calcium. Many green, leafy vegetables are rich in calcium such as Bok choy, spinach, kale, mustard greens, chard, etc. You can also get calcium from soy milk, rice milk, almond milk, and hemp milk.

Omega 3 Essential Fatty Acids

Flax seeds, walnuts, soybean, chia seeds are all excellent sources of omega 3 essential fatty acids.

Vitamin B12

If you are Ovo-vegetarian, then you can buy fortified eggs. Many non-meat and non-dairy sources are also rich in Vitamin B 12. Soy and rice milk are also fortified with this B-vitamin. You could consider taking a daily supplement containing 250 mcg of methylcobalamin.

Iron

Iron is found abundantly in green leafy vegetables such as spinach, as well as in beans, lentils, fortified tofu, etc. The key is to take plenty of Vitamin C through lemon or lime juice, strawberries, raspberries, and other citrus fruits, etc. to ensure absorption of iron. Avoid eating calcium rich foods with iron rich foods since the former hinder with the absorption of iron.

Tips For Getting The Most Out Of Your Clean Eating Diet

•Eat iron-rich foods with vitamin C-rich foods.

•Cook the food in cast iron utensils. Simmering tomato sauce in iron pots can increase its iron content several times over. Likewise, using lemon and lime juice in said pots can also increase the iron content of the food.

•Avoid drinking tea and coffee as the polyphenols in these beverages bind with iron and hinder their absorption.

•Replace eggs with soy, tofu or tempeh.

•Replace chicken with non-GMO tempeh. Tempeh strips can also easily take the place of chicken strips.

•Likewise, replace turkey with tempeh.

•Replace seafood, scallops, etc. with non-GMO tempeh

•Replace eggs with beans, tofu, etc. Vegetarians may use cottage cheese to scramble in place of eggs. Add plenty of herbs, spices and avocados.

•Noodles can easily be replaced with green lentils and mung beans to make a delicious stir fry.

•Add hemp, sunflower, flax and pumpkin seeds to sprinkle over all meals.

In the next chapter, we will discuss plant-based recipes to start your clean eating diet.

Chapter 5: Plant-Based Recipes For A Clean Diet

Let us now discuss some clean eating recipes for seven days. I have included seven breakfasts, seven lunches, seven dinners, and seven snacks. You will find these meals easy to prepare and also healthy and delicious.

Plant Based Recipes

Day 1

Breakfast

Raw Buckwheat Porridge

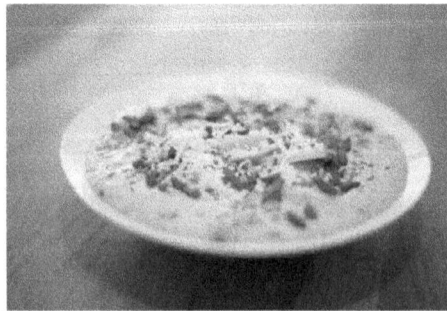

Ingredients

- 1 cup raw buckwheat groats

- ½ cup almond milk

- 1 tbsp Chia seeds

- ½ tsp pure vanilla extract

- 2 tbsp organic natural sweetener (stevia or agave nectar)

- ½ tsp pure cinnamon powder

- Almond slivers, flax seeds or coconut shreds to garnish

Method

- Soak groats overnight in water.

- Next morning, drain the excess water and wipe them dry with a clean kitchen towel.

- Run the groats in a blender or food processor.

- Add almond milk, chia seed, extract, sweetener and cinnamon. Blend for another ½ a minute.

- Scoop in bowls. Serve with fruit, nuts or your favorite toppings.

Snack

Sesame Pita Chips

Ingredients

- 4 pita breads-7 " each

- Sesame oil

- 1/3 rd cup sesame seeds

- Sea salt

Method

- Preheat oven to 350F.

- With a serrated knife, slice open the pita breads into two circles each.

- Coat the breads with sesame oil.

- Cut each pita bread into 8 pieces. Arrange them on a baking sheet, sprinkle sesame seeds.

- Bake for 10 minutes.

•Serve immediately. It can stay for 1 to 2 days at room temperature.

Lunch

Southern Style Corn Black Bean Salad

Ingredients

•3 corn ears husked

•1/3 rd cup pine nuts

•2 tbsp extra virgin olive oil

•Lime juice-1/4 tsp

•Chopped herbs (cilantro, parsley)

•Sea or rock salt and pepper to taste

•30 oz black beans, cooked

•2 cups shredded cabbage

•1 tomato diced

•½ cup minced red onion

Method

•Cook corn by boiling it in hot water. Cut the kernels out with a knife, when cool enough to handle.

- Roast pine nuts in a pan until fragrant.

- In a bowl, mix together oil, lemon juice, herbs, pepper and salt.

- In a larger bowl, add vegetables, beans, corn and onions.

- Add the lemon-oil mixture. Toss to coat.

- You can make this the night before and take it to work.

Dinner

Couscous With Swiss Chard

Ingredients

- Gluten free couscous -10 oz

- ½ cup pine nuts

- 3 tbsp extra virgin olive oil

- 2 cloves garlic

- 15 oz chickpeas (soaked for 8 hours and pressure cooked until soft)

- ½ cup raisins

- 2 bunches of Swiss chard with stems trimmed

- ¾ tsp sea salt

- ½ tsp pepper

Method

- In a bowl, mix 1 ½ cups of hot water with couscous. Cover with a tight lid and let stand for 10 minutes.

- Roast pine nuts until golden brown and fragrant.

- Heat oil in a skillet and add garlic.

- Add chickpeas, raisins, chard, salt and pepper and cook for a few minutes.

- Fluff couscous with a fork. Serve in individual plates. Top with chickpeas and chard and sprinkle pine nuts.

Day 2

Breakfast

Chickpea Omelet With Asparagus

Ingredients

- 8 oz asparagus with stalks trimmed

- ½ cup superfine Chickpea flour

- 2 tbsp nutritional yeast

- 1 tbsp ground chia or flax seeds

- ¼ tsp turmeric powder

- ½ tsp baking powder

- ¼ tsp sea salt

- ¼ tsp pepper

- 1 tsp dried herbs (basil, thyme etc)

- ¾ cup water

- ½ green bell pepper finely chopped

- 1 tbsp chives chopped

- 1 small tomato chopped

Method

- Roast asparagus at 425 F for 10 minutes.

- Mix chickpea flour with water, yeast, chia seeds, turmeric and baking powder. Add salt and pepper as well as dried herbs. Also add in the bell pepper. Whisk to form a smooth batter.

- Add some more water to make into pancake batter consistency.

- In a non stick skillet or cast iron skillet, add some oil. Keep the flame on high until the oil is hot but not smoking. Now lower the heat and add a large spoonful of batter in the center of the skillet. Spread evenly until the batter is thin and circular having about 6" diameter.

•Add the chives, tomato on the top and cover and cook for few minutes. Turn and cook on the other side for a few minutes. Add ½ teaspoon of oil from the sides to make sure the omelet does not stick.

•Add the asparagus stalks on one side of omelet and fold in center to form a semi circular wrap.

•Repeat with remaining batter. Makes two large omelets.

•Serve hot.

Snack

Almonds And Goji Berries

Ingredients

- 20 Almonds

- 20 Goji berries

Method

Mix the nuts and berries together. This ratio has the right amount of sweetness and saltiness. Pack them in your kids' snack boxes and for adults as a healthy clean mid-morning snack.

Lunch

Vegan Gluten Free Burrito Bowl

Ingredients for the burrito bowl

- 1 cup brown rice

- 1 tbsp coconut oil

- Homemade salsa as needed

- Sliced green onions

- Sliced cherry tomatoes to garnish (optional)

Ingredients for the beans

- 2 tbsp olive or coconut oil

- 1 cup onion diced

- 4 cloves of garlic minced

- 1 tsp each chili flakes and dried oregano

- 1 cup chopped tomatoes

- ¼ tsp pepper

- 14 oz black beans cooked

- 2 ½ tsp homemade tomato puree/paste (boil tomatoes, remove skin on cooling and run through food processor)

- Salt to taste

- ½ cup chopped cilantro

Ingredients for the avocado sauce

- 2 cloves of garlic

- 1 large avocado, pitted

- 1 tbsp lemon juice

- 1 tbsp water

•¼ tsp sea salt

Method

•Cook the rice with adequate water and add some vegan butter or coconut oil while cooking. Keep aside.

•To make the beans, take some oil in a skillet. Add the onions and garlic and sauté until golden brown. Add the herbs, tomato paste and beans. Add the salt. Cook until beans are tender. Reduce heat and keep the beans in the skillet on low flame until ready to serve.

•Make the avocado sauce by processing all ingredients in a mini food processor or a small blender. Add little water to ease the process. Taste and adjust lemon juice quantity as desired.

•To serve: divide the rice in 3 bowls. Add beans on top. Add the salsa. Garnish with fresh chopped cilantro, tomatoes and serve immediately.

Dinner

Pineapple Stir Fried Rice

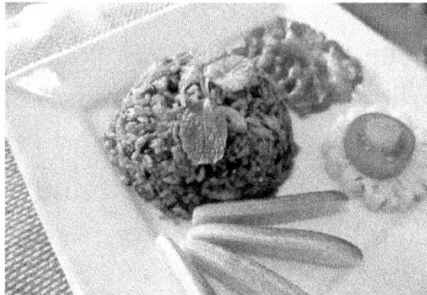

Ingredients

•3 cups brown rice

•3 tbsp olive oil

•2 sliced onions

•4 cups broccoli florets

•4 sliced carrots

•2 diced bell peppers (use all colors)

•6 sliced scallions

•4 tomatoes diced

•3 cups chopped pineapple pieces

- 2 cups coconut milk

- 4 tbsp low sodium soy sauce

- 2 tsp curry powder

- 4 tsp minced garlic-ginger paste

- Cashew, almond slivers and mint leaves for garnish

Method

- Cook rice in a large pan.

- In a skillet, heat oil and add onions and ginger garlic paste until browned. Add the broccoli, carrots and bell peppers. Turn heat on medium and sauté vegetables until crisp.

- Add tomatoes and scallions. Fry for 2-3 minutes.

- Add pineapple chunks. Add the cooked rice and stir gently.

- Add the coconut milk, curry powder and soy sauce. Stir gently to combine all ingredients.

- Serve with nuts as garnish.

Day 3

Breakfast

Mango Smoothie

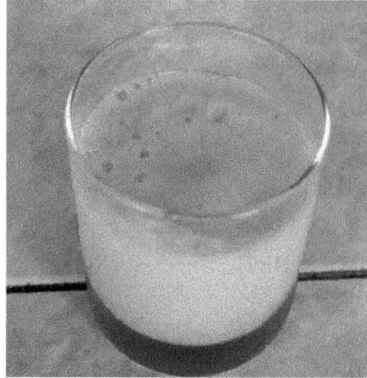

Ingredients

- 1.5 cups fresh orange juice

- ½ to ¾ cups of water as desired

- ¼ cup avocado

- ½ tsp grated lime zest

- 2 cups mango pulp

- Maple syrup to taste

Method

- Blend all ingredients. Enjoy!

Snack

No Bake Energy Bar

Ingredients

- 1 ½ cups Mejdool dates pitted

- 1/3 cup organic unsweetened cocoa

- 1/3 cup chia seeds

- 1 tsp vanilla extract

- 1/3 cup unsweetened coconut flakes

- Pinch of sea salt

- 1/3 cup chopped walnuts

- ¼ cup dark chocolate or chocolate chips

- 1/3 cup oats

Method

- In a food processor, combine the dates, cocoa, chia seeds, vanilla, coconut and salt. Pulse until all ingredients are combined.

- Remove mixture from processor. Add walnuts and coconut flakes. Mix well.

•Take a large wax paper and press the sticky dough onto it. Place the paper with the dough in a square pan and press well in all corners.

•Flip the pan over to get rectangular shaped sticky dough. Wrap in the wax paper from all sides. Refrigerate overnight. Next morning, unwrap and cut into individual bars.

Kale Sweet Potato And Bean Soup

Ingredients

- 1 tbsp olive oil

- 1 medium finely chopped onion

- 3 garlic cloves, minced

- 1 large sweet potato diced in cubes

- 3 cups black beans cooked

- 14 oz. diced tomatoes

- 4 cups homemade vegetable broth

- 1 tsp each of ground cumin, ground coriander and paprika

- 6 cups steamed chopped kale

- 3 tbsp chopped cilantro

- Sea salt and pepper to taste

Method

- Heat oil in a large pot. Add onion and sauté for 5 minutes.

•Add garlic and cook for 1 minute.

•Add sweet potatoes, beans, tomatoes, spices. Fry for a minute.

•Add the broth and salt and pepper.

•Bring mixture to a boil and then simmer for 20 minutes.

•Add kale and cilantro.

•Cook for another 10 minutes or until vegetables are soft. Serve hot with Ezekiel bread.

Dinner

Quinoa With Edamame And Oranges

Ingredients

•2 cups raw quinoa rinsed

•2 tbsp olive oil

•2 cups frozen edamame thawed

•2 medium bell peppers cut in strips

•12 sliced stalks of bok choy

•6 sliced scallions

•2 tsp sesame oil

•3 tbsp low sodium teriyaki sauce

•2 tsp grated fresh ginger

•Pepper

•4 mandarin oranges cut in sections

•1 cup toasted cashew nuts

Method

•Cook quinoa in 3 cups of water. Bring to a boil, then simmer for 20 minutes.

•In a pan, add oil, add the thawed edamame, bell pepper and stir fry for 3 minutes on high.

•Add scallions, bok choy and fry for 3 minutes more.

•Add the quinoa and sesame oil.

•Add pepper, ginger and teriyaki sauce.

•Serve hot by garnishing with orange sections and cashews.

Day 4

Breakfast

Whole Wheat Muffins

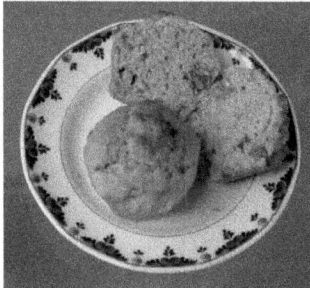

Ingredients

- 1 ½ cups whole wheat pastry flour

- ½ cup stevia

- ¼ cup each of chopped walnuts and raisins

- 2 tsp cinnamon

- Hint of nutmeg

- 1 tsp each baking soda and baking powder

- Pinch of salt

- 1 and ½ cup unsweetened apple sauce

•1 cup shredded carrot

Method

•Preheat oven to 350F.

•Mix all dry ingredients. Then mix the wet ingredients.

•Combine wet and dry ingredients. Mix gently to combine.

•Spoon batter in lined muffin trays. Bake for 20 minutes.

Snack

Spicy Roasted Chickpeas

Ingredients

•1 cup dry chickpeas soaked in adequate water overnight.

•Juice from half a lemon

•1 tsp each of garlic powder, chili powder, cumin powder and curry powder

Method

•Preheat oven to 390 F.

•Put chickpeas in a bowl. Add lemon juice, spices and mix well.

•Place the coated chickpeas on a baking tray lined with baking paper.

•Bake for 45 minutes.

Lunch

Cauliflower Pilaf Recipe

Ingredients

•1 ½ tbsp olive oil

•3 cloves of garlic minced

•1 small cauliflower cut into florets

•3 cups cooked brown rice

•1/3 cup raisins

•1 tsp curry powder

•1 tsp cumin powder

•1/4 tsp cinnamon powder

•3 scallions sliced

•Chopped cilantro to garnish

•Salt pepper to taste

•Red pepper flakes to garnish optional

•Toasted sesame seeds to garnish

Method

•Heat oil in a skillet. Add garlic and sauté.

•Add cauliflower and ¼ cup water to prevent burning. Cover and cook cauliflower until tender.

•Add ginger, rice, raisin, spice powders, and mix well. Cook uncovered for few minutes.

•If mixture is dry, add some water.

•Stir cilantro, scallions and pepper flakes and mix gently. Turn off heat.

•Serve with toasted sesame seeds and cashews.

Dinner

Black Bean Chili

Ingredients

•3 sweet potatoes

•2 tbsp virgin olive oil

•1 cup chopped onion

•2 minced garlic cloves

•1 diced bell pepper

•2 cups cooked black beans

•1 cup diced tomatoes

•1 chopped green chile

•2 tsp ground cumin

•1 tsp oregano

•¼ cup cilantro

•3 sliced scallions

•Salt and pepper as per taste

Method

•Bake sweet potatoes until firm. Cool, dice into cubes and set aside.

•Heat oil in a pan. Add garlic, onions, and sauté until brown.

•Add remaining ingredients except sweet potatoes. Simmer and cook for 15 minutes.

•Cover and cook for another 15 minutes.

•Add sweet potatoes and cook for 15 more minutes.

•Add cilantro, scallions, salt and pepper. Mix well and serve hot.

Day 5

Breakfast

Easy Gluten Free Overnight Pancakes

Ingredients

• 1 cup gluten free flour

• 1 cup chickpea flour

• 2 cups water

• 1 tsp vanilla

• Berries and shredded apples

• Pinch of cinnamon

• 1 tbsp Stevia

Method

• Combine flours and mix with water. Make sure there are no lumps. Cover the bowl with a plastic wrap and leave overnight at room temperature.

• Next morning, heat skillet. Spray a little cooking oil spray and make pancakes.

• Cook pancakes on medium heat until golden brown.

•Serve with fruit and maple syrup.

Snack

Sweet Potato Fries

Ingredients

•3 large sweet potatoes cut in strips/wedges

•1 tbsp olive oil

•1 tsp cumin, 1tsp paprika

•Pinch of cayenne pepper

•½ tsp salt

Method

•Preheat oven to 400 F.

•Place sweet potato strips in a bowl. Add oil, and sprinkle all spices, salt and seasoning. Mix well to coat.

•Place the wedges on a baking sheet and bake for 30 minutes.

Lunch

Easy Peasy Sandwich

Ingredients

•1-2 tbsp Vegenaise (or any eggless sandwich spread without preservatives)

•Homemade chili sauce (grind together a handful of green chilies with an inch of ginger, few cloves of garlic and little water)

•2 slices Ezekiel bread

•Baked tofu

•½ Avocado

•Sauerkraut

•1 tbsp olive oil

Method

•Spread vegenaise and chilli cause on the bread slices.

•Add tofu, avocado and sauerkraut.

•Heat oil in a skillet. Toast the sandwich carefully until both breads are crispy and golden brown.

Dinner

Brown Rice Risotto

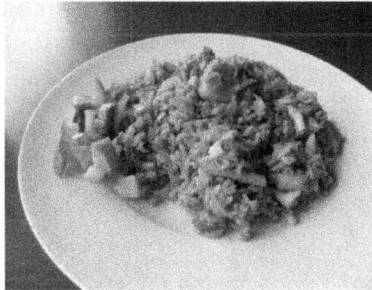

Ingredients

•5 cups vegetable broth (more or less)

•1 tbsp almond butter or coconut oil

•2 tbsp olive oil

•Half red onion finely chopped

•Garlic cloves 2, minced

•1 pinch of red pepper flakes

•1 tsp oregano

•1 tsp fresh thyme minced

•1 tbsp nutritional yeast

- 1 cup brown rice

- ½ tbsp grated vegan cheese

- ½ tbsp grated vegan parmesan cheese.

- Sea salt to taste (if broth does not already have sodium)

- Fresh ground pepper

Method

- Simmer the broth in a large saucepan. Keep it warm while you start your risotto.

- In another saucepan, heat some oil, and add onions. Sauté till brown, about 8 minutes.

- Add the garlic, seasoning, yeast and rice. Let it toast.

- Add I spoonful of broth to the pan, and let it get evaporated. Repeat the step until all the liquid is absorbed, stirring over and over.

- Continue to cook until the rice is creamy. This will take approximately 20-30 minutes. The rice will need about 4 to 5 cups of broth.

- Add the cheeses and mix until combined.

- Add the almond butter or coconut oil.

- Season with salt and pepper.

•Serve with salad and Ezekiel bread.

Breakfast

5 Minute Breakfast Smoothie

Ingredients

•1 cup almond milk

•1 ripe banana sliced

•1 cup fruit of your choice (berries, mango, papaya etc)

•1 tbsp coconut oil

•1-2 tbsp chia seeds

•1/2 tsp grated ginger or 1 tsp powder ginger

Method

Blend all ingredients in a blender until pureed and enjoy immediately.

Snack

Zucchini Chips

Ingredients

•3-4 large zucchinis

•Chopped fresh dill-one bunch (or you could use sundried tomato paste, chili or other natural flavors)

•1 freshly squeezed lemon juice

•A pinch of rock/sea salt

Method

•Using a mandolin, slice the zucchini thinly.

•Spread the slices and apply lemon juice and dill. Mix well to coat the slices evenly. Add a pinch of salt- the slices will shrink after baking so you do not want to over season them.

•Ideally these are made in a dehydrator where they take 24 hours to get crispy. Not all of us have one, so I simply bake them in the oven. If you are using an oven, you must brush the zucchini slices with olive oil.

•Bake at 225 F for 2 hours or until the slices are crispy. Serve after cooling. Store the chips for up to 3 days in an airtight container.

Lunch

Lentil Falafal Salad

Ingredients for Falafals

- 1 cup red lentils

- 2 cups each chopped parsley and cilantro

- 5 cloves of garlic

- 1 chopped red onion

- 1-2 serrano peppers

- 1 ½ tbsp sesame paste/tahini

- 1 ½ tbsp olive oil

- 1 tsp sea salt

- 1 tsp each ground coriander and ground cumin

- 1 to 3 tbsp chickpea powder or spelt flour

- Olive oil spray

Ingredients for tahini dressing

- 1 tbsp Tahini paste

- Juice of 1 lemon/lime

- 3 tbsp water

- 1 clove of garlic grated

- ¼ cup parsley

- ½ tsp paprika

- Salt-pepper

Ingredients for salad

- 3 cups shredded Kale, lettuce, spinach leaves

- 1 grated carrot

- ¼ cup thinly sliced onions

- 3 tbsp olive oil

- 1 tbsp lemon juice

- Sea salt-pepper to taste

Method

- Soak lentils in water overnight.

- Next morning, strain the lentils and pulse them through the food processor until coarsely ground.

- Add the herbs, spices, seasoning, and pulse for few more minutes.

- Drizzle in the tahini paste, oil and blend until smooth.

- Do not over blend-you want a crumbly texture.

•Add baking soda and chickpea flour little at a time. Do not add too much flour as the falafels will become dry. The batter should be fairly moist.

•Refrigerate the mixture for at least 1 hour.

•When ready to make falafels, preheat oven to 375 F. Make round balls of the mixture and place them on parchment paper lined baking tray. Bake for 18 minutes. Do not over bake as they become dry.

•To assemble the salad: Place the falafels on a bed of carrot-lettuce-kale and other salad ingredients. Drizzle with tahini sauce. Add the olive oil on top. Serve immediately.

Cauliflower Butternut Squash Gratin

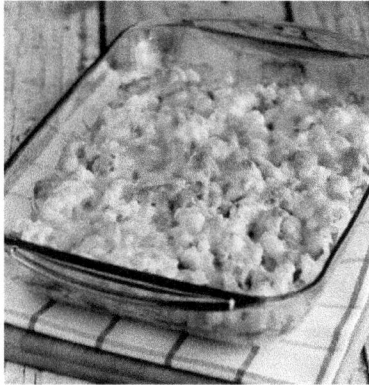

Ingredients

• 1 medium cauliflower cut into florets

• 1 cup corn

• 15 oz of chickpeas cooked

• 1 jalapeno chopped

• 2 tbsp sun dried tomatoes chopped

For the sauce

• ¼ cup cashews

- 1 ¾ cup butternut squash cooked

- 2 tbsp olive oil

- 2 cups almond milk

- ¼ cup coconut cream

- ¼ cup nutritional yeast

- 1 tbsp lemon juice

- 2 tsp each curry powder, onion powder, dry ginger powder, garlic powder (if using ginger garlic fresh, use ½ tsp each grated)

- A pinch of nutmeg

- A pinch of cayenne pepper

- Salt and pepper to taste

Method

- Preheat oven to 400 F.

- In a blender, add all sauce ingredients and puree until smooth.

- In a baking pan, place the vegetables and pour the sauce and mix well.

- Cover with a foil and bake for 30 minutes.

Breakfast

Sweet Pumpkin Caribbean Cornbread

Ingredients

•2 cups grated pumpkin

•2 cups fine coconut powder

•1 cup cornmeal

•4 tbsp almond butter

•1/3 cup coconut sugar

•1 tsp vanilla extract

•½ tsp each cinnamon and nutmeg powders

•Pinch of sea salt

•1 cup warm water

Method

•Preheat oven to 350 F.

•Line a bread pan with parchment paper.

•In a bowl, mix the butter with cornmeal and mix until you get a crumbly texture.

•Now add pumpkin, coconut powder and coconut sugar.

•Mix spices, salt and vanilla.

•Add a little bit of warm water and mix gently. Do not over mix. The bread dough should be dense and not watery.

•Spoon the dough in a baking pan and bake for 45 to 60 minutes.

•Cool completely before slicing.

Beets With Dill & Dairy-Free Cheese

Ingredients

- 1-2 beets sliced thin

- Dill –one bunch, chopped finely

- 1 cup raw cashews

- ½ cup lemon juice

- 2 tbsp nutritional yeast

- Pinch of sea salt or rock salt

- 1 tbsp ground black pepper

- 1 garlic clove chopped

- ½ cup water

Method

- In a food processor, add all ingredients other than beets and dill.

- Add very little water to get thick creamy cashew cheese.

•Once you have the right consistency, add the chopped dill.

•Mix with a spoon.

•Serve on beet slices. Sprinkle some more dill for garnish.

Lunch

Portobello Mushroom Steaks With Polenta

Ingredients for mushrooms

•4 Portobello mushrooms

•Pinch of smoked salt for BBQ flavor

•Pepper

•Coconut oil

•1 tbsp balsamic vinegar

Ingredients for the Polenta

•2 cups corn grits soaked for at least 4 hours

•6 cups water

•4 tbsp Almond butter

•Sprig of un-chopped rosemary

•2 tsp sea salt

•3 tbsp nutritional yeast

•Balsamic vinegar and rosemary for garnishing

Method

•Ina pot, add 6 cups of water, soaked grits and simmer on low heat. Add the rosemary sprig to the pot. Keep stirring to avoid burning at the bottom.

•Continue cooking for 10 minutes. Add the almond butter and yeast and cook until all the liquid is absorbed. Turn off the heat and keep covered until your mushrooms are done.

•Season the Portobello mushrooms with oil and vinegar. Heat the grill and place the prepared mushroom caps on it. Add some more balsamic vinegar on top.

•Let the mushrooms grill on both sides for 3-4 minutes each and drizzle some more vinegar as needed.

•Once done, remove from grill and slice into steak like pieces.

•Serve on the bed of polenta. Garnish with vinegar and rosemary.

Dinner

Easy Veggie Pot Pie

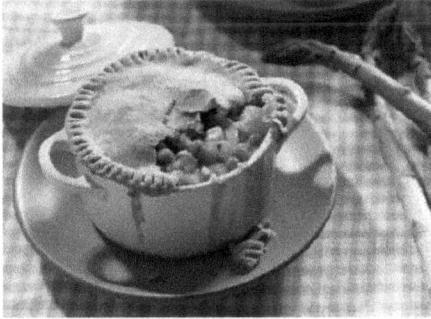

Ingredients for filling

•Vegetables of your choice-1 large potato peeled and chopped, 1 large carrot peeled and chopped, 1 stalk celery chopped fine, 1 medium onion chopped finely, and 1/3 rd cup chopped broccoli florets.

•4-5 mushrooms chopped

•1/3 rd cup each frozen corn and peas

•6 cloves of garlic chopped

•1 tbsp corn starch

• A pinch of sea salt

•1 tsp dried oregano

- 1 bay leaf

- Pinch of red pepper flakes

- 2 cups of vegetable broth

Ingredients for the crust

- ¾ cup each of rice flour and amaranth flour.

- ¼ cup of potato starch plus 2 tbsp

- 1 tbsp arrowroot

- A pinch of salt

- 3 tbsp each of coconut and olive oils

- 1 ½ tbsp of raw unfiltered organic apple cider vinegar

- 2.5 tbsp cold water

Method

- For the filling, sauté the veggies in a skillet.

- Add broth or water and corn starch. Add the bay leaf, oregano, salt, pepper, chili flakes. Stir occasionally until the filling is thick. Remove the skillet from heat. Remove the bay leaf before filling up small sized baking dishes 1/4th full with the filling.

- For the crust-pre heat oven to 350 F. In a bowl, take amaranth, white rice flour, potato starch, salt and arrowroot. Add oil, water, apple cider vinegar, and mix well until you can shape the dough in cohesive ball.

•Roll out the dough on a clean, lightly floured surface. Cut out circular shapes of the dough about ¼ thick and having diameter equivalent to your baking dishes. Place the dough circles on top of the filling on the serving dishes. Press gently to cover and using a fork, press round the edges to create a wave. Coat the top of the dough with olive oil. Bake at 350 F for 25 minutes until the surface is cracked and golden brown.

Chapter 6: Mindfulness And Minimalism

"Be content with what you have; rejoice in the way things are. When you realize there is

nothing lacking, the whole world belongs to you." ~Lao Tzu

Before my family took up the clean living path, we had a lot of stuff: household stuff, toys, books, clothes, workshop stuff and so on. We needed a bigger room to keep all the stuff, so we needed a bigger house. We moved twice and that was also the time my weight ballooned.

After my meditation course, I realized the futility of materialistic desires. Having desire, to an extent, is good, but too much desire leads to negativity, stress and anger. One day, while cleaning the house, we realized we had not used many of the things we had bought in over three years. It was not just financial implication of this realization- I also realized how harmful it was to the environment. Stuff like electronic goods pile up in our over-exhausted landfills and there seems to be no end to the matter.

We started questioning our lifestyle. We decided the excess had to go. We donated large amounts of goods to charity and furniture to goodwill. We recycled items we could not find a home for.

It was not easy. Just like the kids, we grownups were also attached to our things. I kept convincing myself that every item had a memory, a need, a sentimental value attached to it. But the reality remained: I had not used many of those things in over three years. Chances were I would not ever use them again. So we stuck to our plan and continued to purge.

In time, cleaning the home of unwanted things started to become cathartic- it was like a weight being lifted from the shoulders. Our minimalist home soon became clean and this, in turn, reduced the cleaning time I would normally spend on it. We started using the time for taking nature walks. We shifted to a smaller home last year and it is much smaller but a lot closer to the whole foods store, work, library and school.

I had heard of the term Minimalism a couple of times before but it wasn't until recently that we started living like one. I still say to my husband that we are minimalists by accident. He agrees and we both believe that we are happier in the clean living clean eating and simple lifestyle.

Practical Steps To A Clean Minimalist Home

Here are some practical steps to a clean minimalist home:

•De-clutter-one step at a time

It can be overwhelming if you try and get rid of everything all at once. Start small just as you did in case of cleaning your pantry off artificial foods. Begin with the smaller rooms such as the kitchen and bathroom. Before long, you will feel amazing having de-cluttered the room and feel motivated to move to the other rooms.

•Assess the situation

Stand in the middle of the room and ask how you feel. Clutter unknowingly puts pressure and stress on every aspect of our lives. The less clutter you are surrounded with, the better clarity you would have. Take a look around to find items that actually hold meaning in your life. Then remove things that are causing unnecessary stress.

•Simply begin-do not wait

Just begin the purge, do not wait. Place items you find stressful in a box. If needed, sit down for a while with your eyes closed and imagine a minimalist home. Now remove all those items which you did not visualize in the home. If you are moving large furniture items, put them outside the home where they are out of sight. If you have not used an item for more than 3 months, it is time for it to go.

•A place for everything and everything in its place

Teach kids to pick up after themselves. Place each item in its designated spot. Get out of the habit of shoving stuff into closets and cupboards. Assign places according to a purpose. If you are unsure where to place an item, perhaps it does not belong in your clean lifestyle at all.

•Clean

You will find great joy in cleaning a minimalist home. Once a room is de-cluttered, it becomes beautiful and functional. It will eliminate stress, help you find stuff readily and become a place of joy and comfort.

•Stand guard

Unnecessary stuff has a way of finding a way into your home. So stay on guard. Before you buy anything, make sure you really need it. Learn to say no to free samples at malls etc. Let friends and family know you have no need for gifts etc. Instead encourage them to spend time with you. Suggest useful gift items like vouchers, movie tickets or gift cards of stores/restaurants you love.

Stop And Breathe! The Role Of Mindful Breathing In The Clean Lifestyle

Dr. Andrew Weil- Time Magazine's 100 most influential people in 2005 said: "If I had to limit my advice on healthier living to just one tip, it would be simply to learn how to breathe correctly."

Did you know?

The average human breathes 17,000 times per day? How many of us are even aware of our breath? There is also a direct correlation between breath rate (how many breaths an organism takes in one minute) and its lifespan. A dog breathes quite rapidly-at an average rate of 24 breaths per minute. The average lifespan of a dog is 10-13 years. The tortoise, on the other hand, has a breath rate of 4 breaths per minute and lives on an average for 105 years.

Our breath is fast and shallow when we are angry, tense, irritable, or even depressed. It is relaxed, long and calm when we are happier. If our average breath-rate is like that of a dog's we are inviting multitudes of health conditions such as stress, diabetes, heart conditions, etc. Deep, relaxed breathing on the other hand can help bring many multiple positive health benefits including reduced stress, lower blood pressure, better cardiovascular health, and overall improved health.

Just learning to breathe properly-longer and slower breaths can help you lose weight. Do you know how a baby breathes while it is asleep? Its stomach rises and falls with each breath. That is how ideally, we need to breathe. Long, deep and slow.

As we grow older, we forget this ancient knowledge. Our breath gets lost in transition in our materialistic pursuits and busy lifestyles. Society tells us that big bellies are not attractive-so we suck it up and make an effort to look slim. If only we could direct our efforts at our breath, we would automatically correct our posture and reduce weight while preventing lifestyle diseases. So, on the journey of clean eating and clean living, we also need to re-learn the art and science of correct breathing.

Here are simple steps to help you correct your breath and posture:

•Sit or stand comfortably.

•Straighten your neck and back. The spinal column must be straight-so no slouching.

•Place one hand on your stomach and one on your chest.

•Take a deep breath in. While breathing in the stomach should bloat and your hand placed on it should come forward compared to the hand on the chest. As the air enters your lungs, your belly will rise first, then your chest.

•Now start the exhalation. The belly and diaphragm should contract and go inwards.

•You must also learn to pause in between each inhalation and exhalation.

•Do this deep and mindful belly breathing exercise several times a day or each time you feel stressed.

Benefits Of Mindful Breathing

There are many health benefits of mindfulness based breathing.

•Full deep breaths enable your body and mind to relax. This can reduce panic attacks and anxiety.

•Deep belly breathing can help you get in more oxygen in the body. Oxygen is needed for all cells to function properly.

•Breathing slowly, deeply and mindfully can reduce stress. When stress levels are lower, your productivity is higher.

•Your body's immune system functioning is also enhanced. It can counter-attack free radicals which trigger aging, cancer and other diseases.

•When you get angry, practice deep breathing before you say anything. This can help prevent many negative words which can affect relationships. So one of the best benefits of deep breathing is improved relationships.

•Majority of us are seated at our desks everyday hunched over the computers. We rarely give a though to the breath-our life force or Prana. So, simply taking three to four deep long breaths can help replenish this prana to improve focus and mental clarity. If possible, take a walk outside everyday and practice deep belly breathing as explained above.

The science of meditation with breath manipulation is a vast subject. I strongly recommend that you incorporate this in your clean lifestyle. My husband and I attend regular Yoga-Paranyam classes at a yoga studio near our place. If you can do so- it would be great. You will see a dramatic improvement in your health, relationships and productivity at work. If you are working in a high stress environment, take some time to take deep breaths and see how your decision making skills are enhanced!

Mindfulness In All That You Do-Essential Aspect Of Clean Living

Mindfulness means being in touch with your body and thoughts right at this moment. Your mind is not in the past, not in the future but it is completely in this moment. Right Here! Right Now!

When the mind is "here and now", it does not feel fear, pain, hunger, anger, joy or other yo-yo feelings and emotions which it goes through throughout the day. It simply is. This powerful concept can help you stop mindless eating.

Mindfulness is non-judgmental awareness. It involves just observing what our experience is from one moment to the next. It does not judge a moment to be positive or negative.

What is means to be mindful?

•You purposefully pay attention to this moment. You do not judge it as positive or negative.

•You could certainly name the feeling or experience as planning, remembering, sad, happy or worried.

•You allow yourself to just be rather than do or react or change the experience in some way.

•If, during your mindfulness session your mind wanders, you gently bring it to the present moment. You can do this by focusing on the breath.

Activities to do mindfully

•Making your tea or coffee- you do it with complete awareness as if making the tea is the most important thing in the world. See the water boil, then dip the tea bag in it. Watch as the water changes color. Add the lemon. Savor every step of making tea being grateful for having the privilege.

•Washing the dishes. Wash each dish thoroughly. Observe the soap bubbles and watch the water flowing over each dish. Give your complete attention to the process.

•Taking a bath. Touch every part of the body as you do so. Savor the smells, the feeling of your skin. Be grateful for your body. It is a gift to you from Nature. Honor and respect your body.

•Taking a mindful walk. Observe the sensations in your body as you walk. Breathe in slowly and mindfully. Notice the trees, the leaves and breathe in the air. Hear the sounds and noises in the environment. Be in complete harmony with those sounds.

Benefits of mindfulness

•Clarity of thought- What you put into your mind is what will come out of it. When you put in positive and harmonious thoughts, the thoughts that come out also become harmonious. When you practice and make it a habit, the more habitual mindfulness becomes.

•Noticing thoughts helps you drop unwanted thoughts- When you start practicing mindfulness daily you will learn to drop negative thoughts. You drop negative self talk that leads you to destructive habits. For example, if your body tells you to eat, your mind will observe the hunger. As you get into the observe-only-mode, you do not react by eating mindlessly. You also stop as soon as you are full.

•It is like weight training for the mind- Mindfulness is to the mind what exercise and weight training is for the body. It can help increase mental strength to help you tide through any situation. Our mind normally has the habit of telling you to think negative and spiral out of control. But through mindfulness meditation, you learn to stop the train of thoughts and direct them where you want them to go instead of them taking you to where you do not want to go.

•Decreased chronic pain- Research has shown that mindfulness meditation can help reduce fibromyalgia pain and distress.

•Improved sleep- Practicing meditation daily can improve sleep quality, help reduce dependence on sleep medication and help you sleep faster and longer.

•Eating disorders- Mindfulness meditation can be used for treating binge eating and also increase eating self-efficacy.

•Smoking cessation- Many smokers and substance abusers have given up their habit with the help of meditation.

Slow down!

Our society today is over busy and over stimulated. It contributes to restlessness and feeling of depletion, compulsion and overwhelm. We are trained to multitask. We do not enjoy the task at hand, simply because we are feeling pressurized to move to the next task.

Instead of human beings, we have become mechanical robot like creatures that simply cannot rest. We are not allowed to rest since resting is looked down upon as laziness. Going slow in this society means goings against the grain. But it is time we slow down. Accept your body and your limitations. You can change through the process of awareness and acceptance. Face your life as it is with full gratitude, gentleness and joy.

Congratulations, you noticed! You can now begin your clean eating, clean thinking and clean living journey!

Chapter 7: A Scientifically Proven Method Of

Losing Weight Fast And Getting Healthy

In this chapter, I want you to talk about proven steps and strategies on how to make the best of a detox program that scientists and common people worldwide wholeheartedly recommend. It is called Intermittent Fasting.

The reason why both medical researchers and people who use intermittent fasting to lose weight are so enthusiastic about it is simple. There is solid and extremely reliable evidence that indicates the power of intermittent fasting not only for sure and fast weight loss but also for numerous other positive effects on your health that you can notice after a while.

Intermittent fasting can work magic on your body and the practical and scientific go hand in hand to support this amazing method. Intermittent fasting is not part of someone's business plan or a random weight loss method that has worked for one or two body types and people only. It is a highly trustable and sophisticated detox program with multilayered benefits. It would be a pity not to take advantage of them!

Here I will introduce you to the basic principles and gains of intermittent fasting while recommending which fasting style can work best for you. I will try to present this program in its whole complexity and help you choose what is most suitable to your lifestyle, age, health condition, and purpose. Intermittent fasting is, after all, a rather flexible, but incredibly powerful method for losing weight, staying fit, and gaining myriad other bonus benefits for your health and beauty.

You have to understand why you shouldn't ignore the value of intermittent fasting and how you can quickly and easily implement it into your life. Practicing intermittent fasting doesn't feel like a nuisance, sacrifice, or strict regimen. You can very smoothly assimilate it as a highly constructive and healthy eating routine. After all, that's the paradox of intermittent fasting: you can merely eat with breaks and your weight loss is guaranteed.

What is intermittent fasting and how effective is it?

Nowadays there are myriad weight loss methods and full programs that people can try and share with others. And yet many of us find ourselves in an impasse because we either don't know what to choose to make sure it works best for us, or we notice there are differences from one person to another.

Have you ever found yourself dissatisfied with the advice of a friend when you noticed what works for them proved to yield little or no results in your case?

Unfortunately, it's not your friend's fault — it's just a fact of medicine and biology. Our bodies have their own methods of staying fit and regulating their own processes and, if we're lucky enough, we may come across what's optimal for us quite fast.

What if we don't and we keep trying various diets that promise to get us rid of unwanted pounds, require time and effort for preparing the praised food, but don't prove too effective or worthwhile?

Such things have surely already happened to you and you're probably wondering if you personally did something wrong when you were on a specific diet. So how do you get out of the "weight rut"? How do you find an effective method or item that can truly help you lose weight? Needless to say, it's quite important for many of us to lose weight fast and to stay fit even after finishing a given diet or weight loss program. Of course, if you start wolfing anything you can as soon as you finished your diet, you won't be able to keep your desired weight.

However, if you are very careful about what you eat and you lead an appropriate lifestyle that also involves movement, reaching your desired weight and maintaining it is totally possible.

Has anybody found a solution for such problems we all come across when we want to lose weight? Intermittent fasting certainly is an exceptional method!

So what is it about and why is it different from actual diets?

First of all, intermittent fasting is rather a holistic detox practice by means of which you can also lose weight. It's not exactly a diet and yet much more than a diet. How come? Intermittent fasting doesn't "force" you to eat only particular kinds of food, limited quantities, or specific food combinations in order to lose weight. What does intermittent fasting actually mean? Well, as the name already tells you, it's a program that implies not eating … for specific time intervals or according to well-defined plans and programs.

While fasting usually has religious connotations in most cultures, scientists have started to support this program for various purposes. For instance, Walter D. Longo and Mark P. Mattson are only two researchers who dealt with intermittent fasting and underlined its formidable contribution to health and fitness.

Many scientists inform us about the amazing role that intermittent fasting can play in obesity reduction, prevention and reversal of oxidative damage and inflammation, improvement of energy metabolism and others. As such, intermittent fasting is one of the most powerful programs for weight loss, slowing of aging processes, muscle building, and toning, and even cure for specific diseases. How could you not consider all these benefits and include intermittent fasting in your life?

Fasting literally means ingesting no food. Does it also mean starving? That's actually one of the most interesting paradoxes of intermittent fasting: if you fast for limited intervals, you won't really starve! There's little danger to intermittent fasting if done wisely and moderately. The irony is that you will feel a sensation of hunger only initially. After a while (a number of hours or a day, depending on the type of fasting you choose), the hunger one would normally expect will disappear.

So under these rather funny circumstances why not try fasting? You will not have to suffer. For some reasons which are both psychological and physiological, a low-calorie diet or one based on one type of food only (e.g. the daily dissociated diet) is less effective than intermittent fasting. Eating too little or only fruit all day long will actually make you feel hungry. Well, believe it or not, intermittent fasting seems to have a magical side to it. Not only does it protect you from uncomfortable and imperative hunger, but also it helps your body regenerate.

Initially used in various religions as a way of showing self-sacrifice as well as purging the body, fasting is now acknowledged as a medical method with myriad benefits. People are monitored in many clinics as they undergo a period of fasting. Did you know that fasting can last even one week or longer? If you want or have to adopt a "harsher" program, it's always advisable to only do this under medical care and supervision.

However, you can manage milder forms of fasting on your own. Let's see why you should definitely practice fasting!

Intermittent fasting offers you the chance to regenerate your cells apart from being a fantastic means of regulating weight. Intermittent fasting is also more and more appreciated after scientists discovered a relation between our ancestor's longevity and their (often involuntary) lifestyle.

Our ancestors sometimes had to live in forms of scarcity and not eat anything for a day or two. Even unintentionally, this proved to have a good effect on their health. Intermittent fasting activates a significant process in our body, namely cell repair. It reduces oxidative stress and detoxifies the whole body. Implicitly it also helps us lose weight, as one would expect: if you don't eat for one day or more, you only burn calories without adding others into your body.

However, it's essential to understand what a smart and effective way of losing weight intermittent fasting is. Why? Well, it all comes down to the fact that this method naturally involves fast "burning" first of all. While you fast, before your body starts "feeding on" your own muscle, it "eats" your undesirable mass, namely fat. Isn't that simply amazing?

The whole mechanism starts from a protection device of our bodies when faced with the need to go on no food for a while. When food is not available, your body starts using its own cells to feed on. Although this sounds like a magical trick or something purely metaphoric, at the core of intermittent fasting and its superior efficiency lies a very intelligent and powerful organic process.

The first thing your body automatically feeds on to survive is your "bad" cells. Does one have such cells? We all do: they can be damaged cells, tissue affected by forms of disease, older cells, and last, but not least, fatty tissue. As such intermittent fasting is a real boost for your whole body and its natural regenerative processes.

Intermittent fasting is a wonderful genetic repair mechanism that people should use not only for fast weight loss but also in order to stay healthy and young for a longer time. It will help you destroy your degenerated, useless, or unwanted cells. Even cancer cell formation and proliferation can be prevented this way. Intermittent fasting also stimulates the release of the growth hormone, which enhances cell regeneration.

What You Have To Know About Intermittent Fasting
Before You Start Practicing It

Fasting can be as easy or difficult as your body allows for and as you wish. Keep in mind modern science, especially when geared mainly towards weight regulation, also includes regular meal skipping among forms of fasting.

However, if you need a stronger method of weight control or you want to benefit from considerable health improvement as well, it's most recommendable to go for a longer fasting interval. The key is keeping it regular and smartly alternating fasting with "normal" eating habits. That's why it's called intermittent fasting after all and not merely "fasting"!

It is an efficient event if you fast 24h per week or every two weeks. This could be your "maintenance ritual". Nevertheless, when fasting has so many amazing results, you should keep in mind that it's best to fast at least 2 days in a row. Why? Nobody wants you to starve, don't forget this! The reason why has a solid medical basis. Weight loss and cell regeneration are driven by a process called ketosis that only has a full effect after 48-72 hours of refraining from food.

Ketosis inhibits the production of insulin, stimulates the release of the human growth hormone, and promotes the partial destruction of bad, useless, or damage cells. Think of fasting as the best way to destroy your "weakest" cells without suffering yourself.

Most people who haven't tried intermittent fasting yet are worried they will feel hungry and unable to function when they don't eat. While there are a few factors to consider when you fast, this program is by no means extremely difficult.

Humans can easily survive without food for a few days and even weeks, if vitamins and nutrients levels in their bodies are high enough. This is one of the most important aspects you should take care of before embarking on intermittent fasting, especially when you want to go without food for longer than a half day. Ideally, you should eat very diverse food in moderate to high amounts before you start a more intensive fasting program. You don't have to stuff your own body with food when you actually want to lose weight! The point is avoiding to start fasting right after you've tried a low-calories, low-protein, or dissociated diet.

Before you start fasting, go to some specialists for blood investigations and check the levels of vitamins and nutrients in your body. If you fast for longer periods (e.g. several days), you should also take supplements as you fast.

So can you really fast this way? Does fasting mean ingesting absolutely nothing? Actually, intermittent fasting should only mean living on no food while drinking certain types of liquid to keep your body hydrated. Many people recommend water fasting, especially for weight loss. You should actually drink plenty of water. The ideal quantity is 2-3 liters per day.

However, you can also resort to other types of drinks as long as they don't add many calories into your body and they can help you feel invigorated. You can drink your tea of choice as it will only benefit you. Coffee is also allowed, in case you cannot live without it and you need your regular mental energy. By no means should you consume coke, energy drinks, or other beverages full of additives and calories.

Ideally, you should exclude alcohol from your daily drinks while you are on intermittent fasting. Maybe one glass of natural red wine or a bit of cognac won't completely make your fasting counterproductive. However, you will certainly add caloric intake when you want to lose weight. Besides, you will get dizzy and maybe even drunk very quickly if you consume any alcohol while your body doesn't have any food to "chew on". So you'd better forget about alcohol while you are fasting, as this option is the most advantageous regardless of your purposes.

Does fasting have any side effects or things you should be warned against? The truth is it can and thus you have to be very informed before you start practicing it. First of all, a looser method of fasting e.g. skipping 1-2 meals only won't likely affect you in any way.

Stricter and more prolonged programs (starting from one day without food), apart from being distinctly more powerful, will also expose you to a few side effects you should consider. You will feel weaker after 2-3 days of fasting, that's why it's much better to opt for this longer detox program when you are on holidays or simply don't have much workload to manage.

After the 3rd and 4th day, you might be prone to feel a bit dizzy and less energetic. If you want to fast for a few days in a row or one whole week, you should start staying at home or at least spending your time with light activities around your house e.g. in your garden, in a park nearby, visiting a neighbor etc.

You are most likely not going to experience anything serious such as fainting, but it's more comfortable for you to be close to your home if you feel weaker. For instance, the feeling of tiredness and listless might grow after the 3rd and 4th day of fasting, so you will probably feel good if you lie on your bed to rest when you need to.

Do you have to get completely inactive while you fast? Not exactly. It's great if you deal with lighter tasks that don't require maximum concentration power and energy. You can read books you like or need, for instance. Or you can solve problems around the house, perform usual household chores, cook etc. Just avoid fasting for longer than one day when you have to go to work and deal with your regular workload and team.

Your performance might not be optimal due to reduction of energy, nutrients, and caloric intake.

As already mentioned, you will experience a sensation of hunger, especially on the first day. If you are used to eating your breakfast and lunch at specific hours, you might feel the need to keep your eating habit. However, this feeling can be ignored or forgotten, if you simply go about your other activities. By no means will it be insufferable or stringent.

After the 2nd day, your mind and your body will get accustomed to your "newly acquired" eating habits and you will most probably feel no hunger at all during the day. The majority of people who have tried fasting report the fading out of the sensation of hunger after the 1st day.

You might not have to start eating again after 3 or 4 days out of urgent hunger, but your body and brain are prone to feeling the need for more energy and capacity to work properly. For this reason, unless you are under medical care and monitoring, the best way of fasting is stopping after the 5th day maximum. Don't push your limits. You can resume your fasting one week after.

Another important detail to keep in mind is the need to close the fast in a very smooth way. How do you actually close the fast? Actually, the best way is putting it is that you must resume your meals through a very slow and "pure" transition. Your first meal after a period of fasting should be light, nourishing, and healthy. Ideally, you should eat breakfast as your first meal. Eat some very light salad on your first day of eating. Go for fruit and vegetables. These are great ways for making a smooth and inoffensive transition.

One thing to keep in mind is that your feeling of hunger and craving might be strong once you start eating again. For this reason, you have to consciously control your desire and urge and eat very little and light as you close your fasting.

Losing Weight With Intermittent Fasting

Losing weight is quite easy if you practice intermittent fasting instead of a diet. If you can refrain from eating during the first day, the following 2-5 days are not a big deal, since the sensation of hunger slowly disappears. The interval that is most recommended for fast weight loss is 2-5 days. This way you will get rid of kilextra weight and your body will not be affected by side effects.

When you want to lose weight, you can drink plenty of tea made of herbs or spices that are known to accelerate fat burning. For instance, use ginger, turmeric, chili powder, garlic, apple cider, ginseng, green tea, lotus flower tea, rooibos tea etc. Such drinks will help you boost your metabolism, fat reduction, and anti-oxidation processes while adding some more energy into your body and mind.

What should you expect from a few days of fasting? If you are still not fully convinced of the power of this method, you should know that most people report losing ½-1 pounds a day. If you are a person whose body both loses weight and gains pounds easily, you are lucky this time! You can even lose 1 pound a day as you fast. For this reason, intermittent fasting is the most desirable weight loss program when you have to "melt" a few pounds before a specific event such as a wedding, party, presentation etc. It's enough to fast for

3-4 days and you can already be one size smaller. Isn't this extraordinary?

Intermittent fasting is the best means of weight control when you want fast and sure results. It definitely works better than low-calorie diets that ask you to eat very little while feeling hungry and tempted. If you want to take full control of your weight and body, you are welcome to practice intermittent fasting every week (e.g. one day) or every two weeks (3-5 days).

This method is also great when you have gone too far on a certain occasion and have eaten too much or too unhealthy and you don't want your body or your waist to reflect 1-2 pounds more. For instance, after you've eaten all night long at a wedding party, you can simply fast on the next day and you won't put on any weight. You won't feel hungry and lethargic at all, either, since you have stuffed your body with food on the day before.

Intermittent fasting is perfect as a long-term strategy. If you only fast a few days, you will just lose a few pounds. Ideally, you should have your own regular fasting program at least twice a month with the target interval that works best for you and suits your schedule/activities. For example, you can fast for 1-2 days every weekend, when you don't have to work too hard. Alternatively, you can fast 3-4 days every two weeks.

Is this method better than going on a difficult diet for a full month or two weeks? Absolutely. You will help your body get accustomed to this "weight loss and purging ritual" and after a while, you may not even feel any hunger …not even on the first day of fasting. This way you'll also be able to reduce your weight even when it is more substantial.

Through fasting, you can easily and healthily lose even 10 pounds a month or more. The key is keeping track of your nutrient and vitamin intake and levels and having enough discipline, desire, and willpower.

Scientists claim that even intermittent calorie restriction can lead to considerable weight loss. You don't necessarily have to eat nothing at all. You can also just reduce your calorie intake with 15-60% of your usual amount of calories. How can you do this? By skipping one meal, ideally lunch and/or dinner. Most people who don't want to fast for whole days report that they lose weight best when they fast during the second part of the day. You can thus fast for 14, 17, or 20 hours. K. A. Varady supports the method of calorie restriction that spreads on a longer term. In his view, evidence indicated that significant calorie restriction for 8-12 weeks can result in important weight loss – more than if you just fast for 1-4 days in a row and then get back to your older eating habits for months.

Different Intermittent Fasting Methods

Some researchers have noticed that omitting breakfast is not recommended and useful for weight loss. You probably already know that many consider it the most important meal of the day. For instance, Hamid Farschi, Moira Taylor, and Ian Macdonald underline that even for the purpose of weight loss omitting breakfast can be counterproductive as it impairs fasting lipids and insulin sensitivity.

Thus, you can see that some scientists support not only the validity of a "session" of intermittent fasting for less than 24 hours but also its high efficiency. If you don't have to discard many kilos quickly or if you have to work while you plan your fast, go for this method as a good maintenance way of fasting with very few to no side effects.

There is evidence that such a method of fasting (for 15-18 hours) is optimal for gaining lean tissue while losing fat. If you want to build muscle or to keep your body toned as you grow older, this is the way to go! If you are prone to feeling weak quickly or have to work a lot while sticking to your weight loss plan, you should definitely choose a mild fasting program that nevertheless implies meal skipping instead of merely not eating anything after you go to bed and while you sleep. Is it difficult? Just think about it: if you have lunch at 2 pm, you can eat again on the next day at 8-9 am. If you don't want to skip any meal, you can simply have dinner at 5-6 pm and then your next breakfast at 9-10 am, lunch at 2pm and so on. This is the easiest fasting form that doesn't affect your social or professional life at all.

You should, however, stick to healthy food and a lower caloric intake, but it's not necessary to literally monitor the last aspect as in a regular diet. Opt for this method if you want to fast regularly on an unlimited long term without going too hard on yourself. This method is extremely easy to implement and follow as an eating-and-weight-loss routine. Eat larger portions if you only want to have 2 or one meal per day.

Another option is the 24h fast that you can follow once or twice a week. Why should you want to choose this one? Because it will allow you to get rid of up to 2 pounds when you need to, even after some excess. If done regularly, it can help you lose 2-4 pounds per week. Keep this style on a longer run and you can almost imperceptibly and painlessly lose weight even when you are on the overweight side. This program is also recommended by fitness specialists such as Brad Pilon who uses the notion of "Eat.Stop.Eat" to describe it. And this is quite realistic and comforting, as you really won't feel as if you are fasting, but rather intermittently eating.

Use this method when you want to take advantage of a day off and lose 1-2 pound quickly. You are allowed to eat anything and drink low-calorie beverages during your fasting day. Nevertheless, you should be warned against the risk of falling into binge eating with this method. You might be tempted to eat a lot when you're done with your fasting day and regain what you've just lost in a blink of an eye.

The most recommended, but also the most drastic intermittent fasting style requires completely cutting off food for 2-3 days in a row or more. You have to make sure your body has enough vitamins and nutrients already when you start such fasting. Why is this method ideal? On very special scientific grounds: the significant process of ketosis which makes your body start feeding on its own "bad cells" (including fatty tissue) starts after 48-72 hours of fasting. If you want to both lose weight and attain many other health benefits that derive from cell regeneration, go for this method!

You will have to use all your willpower to refrain from eating for 2-5 days in a row, but the positive effects are priceless, even if the first and most obvious thing you can see is considerable weight loss. Think about the value of getting rid of 4-5 pounds at once and put yourself through a test. If you make if to the 4th day once, you can practice this method twice or once a month.

Dr. Joel Fuhrman explains that, once full ketosis is reached, your body loses less weight. Thus, by the 3rd day of fasting, you will be going without food for more far-reaching health benefits rather than for weight loss only. However, this means it's enough to fast for 2-3 days once or twice a month in order to stay fit and lean.

Other Benefits Of Intermittent Fasting For Your Health

After systematic use of intermittent fasting (months to years), you will notice benefits may initially seem to be less realistic or at least quite hidden. First of all, you will feel more energetic and healthy overall, your immunity will improve, and your skin will look much better.

There is no risk of losing muscle if you stick to fasting for 4-5 days. What you will lose is fatty tissue. The principle behind this comes down to a smart mechanism in your body, namely fat/damaged cell burning and protein sparing.

Proteins and amino acids help regenerate cells in our whole bodies as well as in tissue repair. As you keep fasting, collagen helps you improve the condition of your ligaments, muscles, tendons, bones, and last, but not least, the quality of your skin. That's why intermittent fasting is one of the most powerful long-term anti-aging strategies.

Intermittent fasting can even contribute to more serious and dangerous health problems, unbelievable as it may seem at first. Science tells us this holistic detox method can reduce inflammation, accelerate metabolism, reduce cholesterol levels, reverse diabetes, prevent cardiovascular disease, reduce oxidative stress, increase your capacity to fight disease and keep infections and illness at bay as you grow older, decrease blood pressure etc.

Medical scientists also claim that longer-term intermittent fasting (days to weeks) is a good way keeping cancer away or curing it if it is incipient. In case you wonder why, it all comes down to the same cell regeneration principle explained before: damaged/harmful/unhealthy cells are destroyed by your body as it starts feeding on its own tissue, while good cells are protected and their health is enhanced.

Another benefit that you shouldn't ignore is muscle building. Not only does intermittent fasting help you lose fatty tissue, but also it can turn your body into a model of fitness and force, if you practice this program on a regular basis for a long time. It's one of the main means of keeping fit recommended even to athletes, gymnasts, and professional bodybuilders.

Martin Berkhan claims that intermittent fasting is a top method for gaining lean tissue fast whether you lift weights and go to the gym, or you don't work out a lot. It will simply drive your body into a fat-loss-and-muscle-gain working style. This benefit alone is invaluable as you age, so it's a must to practice intermittent fasting!

I hope I was able to help you understand why scientists are so keen on this complex weight loss and health enhancement method. Even if during ancient times people stayed healthy without even practicing intermittent fasting deliberately, modern science helps us realize why it is so effective and how we can use it to stay slim, fit, young, and healthy in the long run without pushing ourselves into harsh, counterproductive, and contradictory diets. Intermittent fasting is better than a regular diet thanks to its safe and sure weight loss results which are accompanied by significant health benefits.

The next step is finding the intermittent fasting style that suits you best and integrate this amazing program of purging your body and keeping healthy into your life. It's actually quite easy: start by fasting for 14-24 hours and you'll find a complete confirmation of the information this chapter introduced you to. Once you realize how easy it is to go on intermittent fasting, you won't be able to refrain from practicing it as your main weight loss method on the long run.

Conclusion

In a world constantly searching for the 'magic pill' for sustained weight loss, the Clean Eating lifestyle puts you on the right track to lose weight without asking you to give up the foods you love. Instead, the Clean Eating approach is to help you find foods you love that are also actually great for you.

The practice of clean eating means consuming foods that are closest to their natural state as much as possible. Many dieticians, doctors, athletes, celebrities and personal chefs have adopted this lifestyle. As I said in the beginning, two words describe the Clean Eating lifestyle: acceptance and mindfulness.

When you start accepting your body, you feel grateful for it. You stop putting demands on it, and you love it the way it is. Once there is love, there is respect – so you avoid putting harmful things inside this temple.

The clean lifestyle is not just about food. It does not consist of a simple list of foods and dos and don'ts. Instead, it's a whole new way of thinking and cooking that can transform our relationship with what and how we eat. Personalization is, therefore, an important part of clean eating. We've all heard statements like, "Stay away from gluten-based foods" and "Stop eating sugar forever". Blanket statements like these just never work. What we need is template recipes and healthier alternatives to help us get started and that we can stick with in the long run. This is the main reason why I've included a 7-day meal plan with delicious and nutritious recipes. If you like those recipes, I believe you'll be more likely to experiment and come up with your own clean food plans.

The clean lifestyle can seem confusing in the beginning. A recent study showed that Americans are better at doing their taxes than eating healthfully. If a food or its preparation is unfamiliar to us, it can quickly push us outside our comfort zone. Even the initial enthusiasm of cleaning up our diet and living clean will peter out when we're faced with weeks of meals to prepare. That's why this book focuses on mindfulness. When you practice daily mindfulness, the preparation process will also become a lot easier.

Overweight people all have one thing in common: they're consuming calories, but they are still starving. The baby needs mother's milk, and we are feeding it colas. Today we are bombarded with nutritionally depleted foods. We also are starving emotionally and spiritually.

The way to lose weight is not to struggle against the body. The best way to lose weight is to figure out what the body wants and give it that. Our bodies also understand one form of starvation: physical. But in many cases, you may be starving emotionally – for love, fun, joy, and intimacy. This is where mindfulness meditation and deep breathing come into play. You learn to observe all your emotions as they come and go and accept them while understanding their triggers. As you get deeper into the practice of minimalism and mindfulness, you avoid putting junk into your home and body.

Clean Eating Guide is not a diet book. It is a roadmap to healthier living. With a little planning, a well-stocked kitchen and a mindful resolve, the clean-eating lifestyle can be easily achieved. With every change you make, each day, each week and each month, you'll be eating healthier and thinking clean – for life!

Part 2

Introduction

A typical 21st century work day consists of an early morning, a hot cup of coffee, a flurry of never-ending meetings, a burger and some fries for lunch, more never-ending meetings, and a slow traffic jam just before you get home. This is true for most of us who work extra hard to earn a decent living in a demanding economic environment. Unfortunately, such schedules have negatively affected our eating habits, with most of us unable to commit the time and energy required to eat clean and healthy. Our poor eating habits have predisposed us to many lifestyle diseases, including obesity and heart disease, which are at an all-time high. Processed foods and foods containing unhealthy fats and high carbs have been associated with increased risks of obesity, cardiovascular disease, cancer, diabetes, and osteoporosis.

Eating clean does not necessarily have to be a complicated affair with 7-day meal plans to get healthy. Clean eating can easily mean the addition of whole grains, healthy fats and proteins, fruits and vegetables to your diet without the need to count calories or remove whole food groups from your diet. In this cookbook, you will find tasty recipes to help you discover better health through clean eating.

Why To Eat Clean

To understand the importance and vitality that clean eating wields, we must grasp the underlying principle on which eating clean is based. To keep it short and simple, the idea behind clean eating revolves around reducing and effectively eliminating all processed food from our diet. This encompasses even the packaged 'natural' juice that you but from grocery shops and supermarkets. In other words, clean eating is founded on the ideals of nourishing and fueling the body with nutritious, chemical-free and wholesome foods.

Currently, as we speak, over a quarter of the world's population is on the brink of starvation and the other half is busy spending countless resources to treat self-imposed, lifestyle disorders such as diabetes, gout, and obesity. This imbalance - to some extent - is caused by our insatiable need to process food unnecessarily that is otherwise healthy and delicious in its most natural form. As a result, we've wrecked irrevocable and irreversible serious damage to the mother nature's balance which ensures sustainability. Therefore, by embracing clean eating, you will not only be promoting sustainable living but also boosting your health by sticking as much as possible to raw, unprocessed, organic food.

In comparison to other existing diets, clean eating has a solid connection to Paleo diet which advocates for the inclusion of only wholesome, natural, sugar-and-free ingredients. If anything, clean eating and Paleo diets can be said to be handmaidens in which one follows the other in uniform succession. In addition to this, remember that clean eating principles also advise towards the intake of copious amounts of fresh water daily in a bid to stay hydrated throughout the day as opposed to sipping frothy drinks or packaged soft drinks. And if this is anything to go by, then we have one more reason you should jump on this bandwagon.

Delicious Clean Eating Recipes

Breakfast Recipes

Baked Oatmeal

Serves: 4
Time: 35 minutes

Ingredients:

2 egg whites
½ cup milk
½ tablespoon canola oil
1 ½ cups uncooked rolled oats
½ teaspoon cinnamon
2 tablespoon raw honey
4 tablespoons applesauce, organic

Directions:

Preheat oven to 350F. In a large bowl, whisk the egg whites, applesauce, oil, and milk.
Fold in remaining ingredients.

Spray 9x13-inch baking dish with cooking oil. Spoon oatmeal into a baking dish and bake for 30 minutes. Serve after.

Nutty Banana Pancakes

Serves: 6
Time: 10 minutes

Ingredients:

1 banana, mashed
2 teaspoons oil
3 egg whites
1 cup whole wheat flour
2 teaspoons baking soda
2 tablespoons chopped walnuts or other nuts
¼ teaspoon ground cinnamon
1 cup milk
1 teaspoon pure vanilla
¼ teaspoon salt

Directions:

Mix all dry ingredients in a bowl.
In a separate bowl, whisk the egg whites, mashed banana, milk, and vanilla.
Fold the liquid ingredients into the dry and stir the chopped walnuts. Heat a large skillet over medium heat.

Coat with cooking spray and when hot add ¼ cup batter per pancake.

Cook for 2-3 minutes or until browned. Flip carefully and cook for 1 minute more. Serve while still hot.

Breakfast Quinoa

Serves: 4
Time: 20 minutes

Ingredients:

1 cup uncooked quinoa, rinsed
¼ cup honey
2 cups milk
¼ cup fresh blueberries
¼ teaspoon ground cinnamon
¼ cup chopped almonds

Directions:

Bring the milk to boil in a medium saucepan.
Add the quinoa and reduce heat. Simmer the quinoa
for 15 minutes or until the milk is completely absorbed.
Remove the quinoa from heat and fluff with a fork.

Transfer the quinoa in a bowl and drizzle with honey.
Top with the fresh blueberries and chopped almonds.
Serve after.

Breakfast English Muffins

Serves: 4
Time: 15 minutes

Ingredients:

2oz. Swiss cheese
8 egg whites, whisked
1 teaspoon olive oil
½ cup grape tomatoes, quartered
4 scallions, diced
Salt and pepper, to taste
Additional:
2 English muffins, whole what, split or toasted whole wheat bread

Directions:

Broil the muffins for 2 minutes or until edges begin to brown.
Heat the olive oil in a large skillet. Cook scallions for 3 minutes.
Add the whisked egg whites and season to taste. Cook until the egg whites are set.

Divide the eggs into four equal portions and use to top the broiled muffins.
Finish off with the cheese and tomatoes.
Serve after.

Pumpkin Pancakes

Serves: 4
Time: 10 minutes

Ingredients:

1 ¼ cups whole-wheat flour
1 teaspoon ground ginger
1 tablespoon baking soda
2 teaspoons cinnamon
1 egg
1 cup buttermilk
½ cup pumpkin puree, organic
1 pinch ground cloves
1 pinch ground nutmeg

Directions:

In a bowl, whisk the dry ingredients. In a separate bowl, whisk the egg, buttermilk, and pumpkin puree. Add the liquid ingredients to the dry ingredients and mix until incorporated.

Heat a non-stick skillet over medium-high heat. Pour ¼ cup batter per pancake and cook until bubbles appear on the surface. Flip carefully and cook for 1 minute more.
Serve while still hot.

Like A French Toast

Serves: 6
Time: 10 minutes

Ingredients:

6 slices whole wheat bread
½ cup milk
2 eggs
2 tablespoons honey
4 tablespoons unsweetened applesauce, organic
1 teaspoon ground cinnamon

Directions:

In a medium bowl, whisk all ingredients. Soak bread one slice at the time until slightly absorbed. Gently coat the skillet with cooking spray.

Cook the toast over medium-high heat until browned on all sides.
Serve while still hot, perhaps with fresh fruits.

Crunchy Fruit Breakfast

Serves: 6
Time: 10 minutes

Ingredients:

1 cup blueberries
1 cup seedless grapes
2 cups chopped pears
2 tablespoons honey
¼ cup sunflower seeds
¼ cup sliced almonds
12oz. yogurt
1 teaspoon vanilla paste
4 tablespoons toasted coconut

Directions:

Divide fruits in equal portions between six parfait or dessert glasses. Top fruit with yogurt and drizzle with honey.

Sprinkle with sunflower seeds almonds and toasted coconut.
Serve immediately.

Simple Grits Waffles

Serves: 4
Time: 15 minutes

Ingredients:

1 ¼ cups whole-wheat flour
½ cup corn grits
¾ cup buttermilk
2 eggs, whisked
1 teaspoons baking soda
6 tablespoons cubed cold butter, grass-fed
1 tablespoon honey
2 cups water

Directions:

Bring water to boil over medium-high heat in a saucepot.
Whisk in the grits and bring to boil. Reduce heat to low and cook for 15 minutes stirring often. Stir in the butter and once incorporated, stir in the buttermilk.

Whisk the flour with baking soda. Add the honey.
Stir the flour mix into the grits. Preheat waffle iron and spread 1/3 cup batter per waffle. Cook according to manufacturers directions. Serve while still hot.

Hot Fruit Bowl

Serves: 2

Time: 10 minutes

Directions:

½ cup amaranth grain
½ cup Greek yogurt
¼ cup chopped figs
¼ cup chopped apricots
2 tablespoons chopped dried cherries
2 tablespoons honey
¼ teaspoon cinnamon
2/3 cup water

Directions:

In a saucepan, bring the amaranth, water, and cinnamon to boil.
Reduce heat to medium-low, add the fruits, and simmer for 10 minutes. Remove from the heat. Mix the yogurt with honey in a bowl.

Divide the amaranth fruit mix between 2 bowls and top with the yogurt mix.
Serve immediately.

Spinach Cake Muffins

Serves: 8 muffins
Time: 20 minutes

Ingredients:

1 ½ cups whole-wheat flour
1 cup packed fresh spinach
½ cup unsweetened apple sauce, organic
1 egg
1 teaspoons baking soda
2 teaspoons pure vanilla
½ cup honey
½ teaspoon salt
2 tablespoon vegetable oil

Directions:

Preheat oven to 350F and line an 8-hole muffin tin with paper cases.
In a food blender, combine applesauce, egg, vanilla, honey, and oil.

Process until smooth and transfer into a bowl. Fold in the dry ingredients and stir until combined. Scoop batter into prepared muffin tin and bake for 12-15 minutes.
Serve at room temperature.

Grape Breakfast Sundae

Serves: 2
Time: 5 minutes

Ingredients:

8oz. Greek yogurt
¼ cup granola, gluten-free
½ cup fresh cottage cheese
½ cup halved grapes
2 tablespoons raspberries

Directions:

In a food blender, process the raspberries and Greek yogurt. Transfer in a bowl and add the cottage cheese.

Spoon into two bowls and top with granola and grapes. Serve after.

Lunch Recipes

Red Peppers Stuffed With Couscous And Chickpeas

Serves: 4
Time: 30 minutes

Ingredients:

1 cup whole-wheat couscous
4 red bell peppers, tops off, membranes and seeds removed
1 cup cooked chickpeas, drained and rinsed
1 cup diced dried apricots
1 teaspoon ground cardamom
½ teaspoon hot sauce or chili powder
1 ½ cups vegetable stock, homemade
1 cup minced flat-leaf parsley
1 tablespoon lemon juice

Directions:

Bring the stock to a simmer over medium heat.

Add the couscous and stir. Remove from the heat and place aside for 5-10 minutes or until the liquid is absorbed. Remove the bell pepper top and dice finely. Stir in the couscous.

Add the chickpeas, cardamom, apricots, parsley, and lemon juice. Stuff the peppers with prepared mixture and place in the baking dish. Bake the peppers at 350F for 20 minutes. Serve after.

Tuna Salad

Serves: 4
Time: 10 minutes

Ingredients:

10oz. can light tuna in water, drained
2 tablespoons red wine vinegar
2 tablespoons extra-virgin olive oil
4 hardboiled eggs, sliced
2 tablespoons parmesan cheese, shredded
½ cup chopped green onion tops
4 cups arugula

Directions:

In a bowl, toss tuna with oil, vinegar, eggs, green onion tops, and arugula.

Divide the salad between four bowls and top each with shredded parmesan.

Edamame Salmon Cakes

Serves: 4
Time: 25 minutes

Ingredients:

2 cups cooked flaked salmon
½ cup thawed frozen edamame
1 garlic clove, minced
1 tablespoon chopped cilantro
1 scallion, chopped
2 whole-grain bread slices, toasted and ground
2 egg whites
1 tablespoon minced ginger
Some oil, to fry

Directions:

Line a baking sheet with a parchment paper. In a large bowl, combine all ingredients by order. Mix it up with clean hands. Form four cakes from the prepared mixture and arrange onto a baking sheet. Pop in the fridge for 15 minutes.

Meanwhile, heat the oil over medium-high heat. Add the cakes and cook for 3-4 minutes per side or until browned. Serve while still hot.

Kale And White Bean Soup With A Twist

Serves: 4
Time: 60 minutes

Ingredients:

12oz. kale, stalks trimmed and torn into pieces
30oz. dry white beans, cooked
1 onion, chopped
1 tablespoon olive oil
½ cup whole grain sorghum, uncooked
6 cups chicken broth, low-sodium, homemade
1 teaspoon hot sauce
2 garlic cloves, minced
15oz. diced tomatoes

Directions:

In a saucepot, bring 3 cups chicken broth to boil. Add the sorghum and reduce heat. Simmer for 25 minutes. Meanwhile, heat oil in a separate saucepot. Add the garlic and onion. Cook over medium heat for 5-6 minutes or until tender. Add hot sauce and kale. Cook until kale is wilted.

Mash ½ cup white beans with a fork in a bowl. Add the mashed beans, remaining white beans, tomatoes, remaining chicken broth, and sorghum to kale mix.

Bring to boil over medium-high heat. Reduce heat to medium-low and simmer for 20 minutes. Serve while still hot.

Chicken Salad With Fig Vinaigrette

Serves: 4
Time: 15 minutes

Ingredients:

4oz. cooked and diced chicken breasts
½ pear, cored and sliced
1 radish, sliced thinly
¼ cup pea shoots
¼ cup bean sprouts
For the vinaigrette:
½ cup balsamic vinegar
¼ cup extra-virgin olive oil
¼ cup chopped figs
1 teaspoon finely grated zest
2 tablespoons roughly chopped basil

Directions:

In a food blender, combine all dressing ingredients. Process the ingredients until blended thoroughly. In a large bowl, combine the salad ingredients.

Pour over prepared vinaigrette and toss to combine. Serve immediately.

Zucchini Pad Thai

Serves: 4
Time: 20 minutes

Ingredients:

4 4oz. chicken skinless and boneless chicken breasts,
sliced
3 cups bean sprouts
2 tablespoons sliced green onions
¼ cup chopped peanuts, unsalted
2 teaspoons olive oil, divided
2 eggs
For the sauce:
4 tablespoons tamarind paste
½ tablespoon Sriracha
1 ½ tablespoons reduced-sodium tamari
4 tablespoons low-sodium chicken stock
2 tablespoons lime juice
For the noodles:
2 carrots, peeled
4 zucchinis, trimmed

Directions:

Prepare the vegetable noodles: spiralizer into ribbons
and place aside.
Prepare the sauce: in a bowl, combine all sauce
ingredients. Place aside.

Prepare the chicken: heat 1 teaspoon olive oil in a skillet. Add the eggs and scramble until cooked through. Season with a pinch of salt. Transfer in a bowl. Wipe out the skillet and heat the remaining oil. Add the chicken and cook cooked through. Place in a bowl with eggs.

Add the prepared sauce into the same skillet. Cook for medium heat until slightly thickened. Add the prepared zucchinis and carrots and cook for 5-6 minutes or slightly softened. Add in sprouts, egg, and cooked chicken. Divide the Pad Thai between serving bowls and serve while still hot.

Oven Baked Chicken, Potatoes And Brussels Sprouts

Serves: 4
Time: 40 minutes

Ingredients:

1lb. skinless and boneless chicken breasts, cut into 4 equal pieces
1 onion, diced
3 cups red potatoes, cut into chunks
1 ½ teaspoons dried basil
4 cups Brussels sprouts, trimmed, quartered
2 teaspoons whole-grain mustard
¼ teaspoon garlic
4 tablespoons lemon juice
2 figs, chopped
A handful of fresh basil
2 tablespoons olive oil

Directions:

Preheat oven to 400F. Place the chicken into a baking dish. Process the fresh basil, lemon juice, figs and olive oil until you have a smooth mix. In a bowl, whisk the prepared vinaigrette, mustard, garlic, dried basil and lemon juice. Add the potatoes and Brussels sprouts.

Toss to coat with the dressing and arrange around the chicken.

Drizzle the chicken with remaining dressing mix and sprinkle with diced onions.
Bake for 20 minutes or until chicken is cooked through. Transfer the chicken to a plate and stir the veggies. Continue roasting the veggies for 15 minutes. Serve while still hot with prepared chicken

Beef Stew

Serves: 4
Time: 1 hour 25 minutes

Ingredients:

1lb. beef round steak
1 cup diced tomatoes
½ cup diced mushrooms
½ cup diced white potato
1 cup diced celery stalks
½ cup diced sweet potato
1 teaspoon balsamic vinegar
2 teaspoons canola oil
1 cup trimmed and chopped kale
4 tablespoons red wine vinegar
3 cups low-sodium beef stock, homemade
¼ cup uncooked barley
1 tablespoon dried basil
1 teaspoon dried chopped rosemary
1 cup diced carrot
4 garlic cloves, minced
2 onions, diced
1 teaspoon minced fresh thyme

Directions:

Preheat the broiler and broil the steak for 10 minutes, turning once.

Place aside to rest. Dice after. In a large soup pot, heat the oil over medium-high heat. Add the veggies and cook for 10 minutes, stirring occasionally. Add barley and cook for 10 minutes more.

Add the diced steak followed by stock, vinegar, and herbs. Bring to simmer and cook for 1 hour. Serve while still hot.

Roasted Salmon

Serves: 4
Time: 15 minutes

Ingredients:

4 5oz. salmon pieces, skin on
2 tablespoons chopped chives
2 tablespoons fresh tarragon leaves
4 teaspoons olive oil

Directions:

Preheat oven to 425F and line a baking sheet with foil.
Rub salmon with oil, all sides.
Place the salmon on a baking sheet, skin side down and
roast for 12 minutes or until starts to flake easily.

Lift the salmon off the baking sheet and arrange on a
plate. Discard the skin, sprinkle with the chives and
tarragon.

Stuffed Eggplants

Serves: 4
Time: 35 minutes

Ingredients:

2 medium eggplants, trimmed
½ cup chopped celery
2 cups water
2 tablespoons olive oil
½ cup chopped red bell pepper
½ cup diced onion
4 whole-grain bread slices, toasted and ground
1 cup sliced mushrooms
2 cups chopped tomatoes
12oz. chicken breasts, skinless, boneless and cut into ½-inch wide strips
Black pepper, to taste

Directions:

Preheat oven to 350F and coat baking dish with some oil. Trim the eggplants and cut in half by length. Scoop out the flesh using a spoon, leaving the ¼-inch thick shell. Chop the eggplant pulp and place aside. Place the shells in a baking dish and pour the water around. Heat the olive oil in a skillet. Add the chicken strips and cook for 5 minutes or until chicken is no longer pink.

Add the peppers, eggplant flesh, onion, celery, tomato juice, and mushrooms. Reduce the heat and simmer for 10 minutes. Stir in the breadcrumbs and season with black pepper. Divide the mixture between eggplant shells and if remaining some, place around the eggplants. Cover the eggplants with aluminum foil and bake the eggplants for 15-20 minutes. Serve while still hot.

Dinner Recipes

Polenta With Vegetables

Serves: 4
Time: 55 minutes

Ingredients:

1 cup ground cornmeal
1 cup sliced mushrooms
1 cup sliced zucchini
1 cup sliced onions
1 teaspoon minced garlic
1 cup broccoli florets
4 cups water + 2 tablespoons
2 tablespoons Parmesan cheese, grated
Chopped fresh basil, to garnish

Directions:

Preheat oven to 350F and spray 3-quart baking dish with some cooking oil.

Combine the 4 cups water, polenta, and garlic in a prepared dish.

Bake, uncovered for 40 minutes.

Meanwhile, grease a large skillet with some oil. Heat over medium-high heat and add mushrooms and onions.

Cook for 5 minutes. Add the water, broccoli and zucchinis. Cook for until crisp-tender.

Once the polenta is done, divide between four plates. Top with veggies and sprinkle with the Parmesan.

Serve after.

Provence Pork Medallions

Serves: 4
Time: 15 minutes

Ingredients:

4 4oz. pork tenderloins
½ cup dry white wine

1 teaspoon Herb de Provence
Salt and pepper, to taste

Directions:

Season pork lightly with salt and pepper.

Place the pork between two pieces of parchment paper and pound with a mallet.
You need to have ¼-inch thick meat.

In a large non-stick frying pan, cook the pork over medium-high heat for 2-3 minutes per side.

Remove from the heat and sprinkle with herb de Provence. Remove the pork from skillet and place aside. Keep warm.

Place the skillet over heat again. Add the wine and cook, stirring to scrape down the bits.

Cook until reduced slightly and pour over pork. Serve after.

Chicken And Leek Paella

Serves: 4
Time: 1 hour 10 minutes

Ingredients:

1lb. skinless and boneless chicken tights, cut into ½ - inch thick strips
2 tomatoes, seeded, chopped
1 red bell pepper, sliced
2 cups fat-free, unsalted chicken broth, homemade
2 leeks, chopped, white part only
1 cup frozen peas
3 garlic cloves, minced
1 onion, diced
¼ cup chopped fresh parsley
2/3 cup long-grain brown rice
1 teaspoon tarragon
1 teaspoon olive oil

Directions:

Heat the olive oil in a large skillet over medium-high heat.

Add the chicken, onion, and leek.

Cook for 5 minutes or until veggies is tender.

Add the tomatoes and bell pepper and cook for 5 minutes more.

Add the tarragon and rice and broth.

Bring to boil and reduce heat after. Simmer for 10 minutes. Stir in the peas and simmer for 45-60 minutes or until the broth is absorbed.

Serve while still hot, garnished with parsley and 1 lemon wedge.

Beef With Pomegranate And Cauliflower

Serves: 4
Time: 30 minutes

Ingredients:

1lb. beef tenderloin, fat trimmed
¾ head cauliflower, cut into florets
2 yellow onions, sliced
2 tablespoons olive oil
1 ½ tablespoons lemon juice
4 tablespoons pomegranate seeds
1 ½ teaspoons whole-grain mustard
Salt and pepper, to taste

Directions:

Coat the beef tenderloin with 1 ½ tablespoon olive oil and season with salt and pepper to taste.

Preheat oven to 475F and place the prepared beef tenderloin in a baking dish. Bake for 12 minutes.

Meanwhile, toss the cauliflower with 1 tablespoon olive oil and yellow onion. Season to taste and scatter around the beef tenderloin.

Continue baking for 15 minutes more.

Remove the beef and veggies and place the veggies in a separate bowl. Tent the beef with aluminum foil and allow to rest for 10 minutes.

Whisk the remaining olive oil with mustard and lemon juice.

Slice the beef and arrange onto a plate. Scatter around the veggies and drizzle with prepared sauce. Sprinkle with pomegranate seeds and serve.

Grilled Fajitas

Serves: 8
Time: 20 minutes

Ingredients:

1lb. pork tenderloin, cut into 2-inch long and ½-inch wide strips
1 onion, diced
1 tablespoon chili powder
4 tomatoes, diced
4 cups shredded lettuce
8 whole wheat tortillas, warmed
1 cup salsa
½ teaspoon oregano
½ teaspoon smoked paprika
¼ teaspoon garlic powder
¼ teaspoon ground coriander

½ cup shredded sharp Cheddar cheese

Directions:

Preheat grill to medium-high.

In a small bowl, combine the spices and herbs. Rub the pork strips with the prepared spice mix.

Place the pork strips and onion into a grill basket. Grill for 5 minutes or until browned on all sides.

Spread the equal amount of pork strips and onions on each tortilla.

Top each with 1 tablespoon cheese, tomatoes, lettuce, and salsa.

Fold the tortilla sides over the filling to close. Serve after.

Broiled Bass

Serves: 2
Time: 15 minutes

Ingredients:

2 4oz. sea bass fillets
1 teaspoon minced garlic

1 tablespoon lemon juice
¼ teaspoon herb seasoning blend, sodium-free
1 tablespoon lemon juice
Ground black pepper, to taste

Directions:

Heat the broiler and position the rack 4-inches from the heat source.

Coat a baking sheet with cooking oil.

Sprinkle the garlic, lemon juice, herbs, and black pepper over the fish.

Broil the fish for 8-10 minutes or until opaque.

Serve while still hot.

Chicken Salad With Oranges

Serves: 4
Time: 15 minutes

Ingredients:

4 4oz. skinless and boneless chicken breasts
16 black olives, chopped
2 oranges, peeled and segmented
8 cups lettuce

2 garlic cloves

For the dressing:

1 tablespoon extra-virgin olive oil
1 tablespoon chopped red onion
1 tablespoon chopped celery
4 garlic cloves, minced
½ cup red wine vinegar
Ground black pepper, to taste

Directions:

Prepare the dressing: in a bowl combine the dressing ingredients. Cover and refrigerate.

Prepare the chicken: preheat the grill and lightly coat with oil. Position the rack 4-inches from the heat source.

Rub the chicken breasts with garlic and discard the garlic. Grill chicken for 5 minutes per side.

Transfer the chicken onto a cutting board to rest for 5 minutes.
Slice the chicken into strips.

Divide the olives, oranges, and lettuce between four bowls. Add the chicken and drizzle all with prepared dressing. Toss to combine and serve after.

Five-Spice Pork Medallions

Serves: 4
Time: 30 minutes

Ingredients:

1lb. pork tenderloin, fat trimmed
¾ cup water
4 cups green cabbage, shredded
3 tablespoons dry white wine
½ cup chopped onion
1 tablespoon parsley, chopped
1 tablespoon olive oil
For the marinade:
1 green onion, minced
¾ teaspoon five-spice powder
3 garlic cloves, minced
2 tablespoons low-sodium soy sauce
1 tablespoon olive oil

Directions:

Prepare the marinade: in a bowl, combine all ingredients.

Add pork and turn once to coat. Cover and marinade for 2 hours, turning occasionally.

Preheat oven to 400F.

Remove the pork from marinade and pat dry with kitchen towels.

Heat the olive oil in large skillet and cook pork over medium-high heat for 5 minutes or until browned on all sides.

Add ½ cup water to the pan and place the pan into the oven. Roast the pork until inner temperature reaches 160F. Remove the pork from the oven, place onto a cutting board and tent with aluminum foil.

Place the pan over medium-high heat. Add the wine to deglaze the pan. Add the onion and cook for 1 minute. Add the cabbage and remaining water. Cover and simmer until the cabbage is wilted, for 4-5 minutes.

Slice the pork into 8 medallions. Serve with prepared cabbage, and garnish with parsley.

Serve while still hot.

Mexican Beef

Serves: 4
Time: 40 minutes

Ingredients:

0.5lb. ground beef
2oz. shredded Mexican cheese
½ cup onion, chopped
1 cup bell pepper, diced
2 cups water
2 medium tomatoes, diced
1 cup uncooked rice
2 teaspoon oregano
1 tablespoon chili powder
1 cup frozen mixed vegetables, chopped

Directions:

Brown beef in a large skillet over medium-high heat. Drain fat.

Add bell pepper and onion. Cook for 10 minutes.

Add tomatoes, vegetables, spices, rice, and water. Mix and bring to boil.

Reduce heat to medium-low and simmer, covered for 20 minutes.

Once cooked, divide between serving plates and sprinkle with shredded cheese.

Tandoori Chicken

Serves: 6
Time: 40 minutes

Ingredients:

6 skinless and boneless chicken fillets, cut into ½-inch
pieces
1 teaspoon yellow curry powder
1 cup yogurt
5 garlic cloves, minced
½ cup lemon juice
2 tablespoons paprika
1 teaspoon minced ginger
1 teaspoon crushed red pepper flakes

Directions:

Preheat oven to 400F.

In a food blender, combine yogurt, curry, lemon juice,
garlic, red pepper flakes, ginger, and paprika. Process
until smooth.

Soak the bamboo skewers in a water, and arrange the
chicken onto the skewers in equal portions. Place the
skewers into a shallow dish and pour over the yogurt
mix.

Cover and chill for 15 minutes.

Remove the chicken and arrange onto a baking sheet coated with cooking spray. Discard the marinade.

Brush the chicken with remaining yogurt mix. Bake for 20 minutes or until the chicken juices run clear.

Serve while still hot.

Beverages

Fresh Smoothie

Serves: 4
Time: 5 minutes

Ingredients:

1 cup fresh diced pineapple
1 cup water
1 cup strawberries, hulled
½ cup watermelon, cubed
1 tablespoon honey
-

Directions:

In a food blender combine all ingredients.

Process until smooth.

Serve immediately.

Iced Latte

Serves: 4
Time: 10 minutes + chilling time

Ingredients:

2 cups fresh brewed coffee
1 ½ cup milk
1 cup whipped topping
2 tablespoons honey
2 tablespoons almond syrup
1 teaspoon ground espresso beans
Some ice cubes

Directions:

In a large jug, combine the coffee, milk, honey, and syrup.

Stir well and refrigerate.

Fill 4 glasses with ice. Pour coffee over ice, top with whipped topping and sprinkle with espresso beans.

Orange Delight

Serves: 4
Time: 5 minutes

Ingredients:

4 peeled and segmented oranges
1 cup light vanilla soy milk
1 ½ cups orange juice
1 tablespoon honey
1/3 cup silken tofu
1 teaspoon grated orange zest
Some ice cubes

Directions:

In a food blender, combine all ingredients.

Process until smooth.

Serve immediately.

Green Smoothie

Serves: 4
Time: 5 minutes

Ingredients:

1 cup cold water
1 banana
½ cup strawberries
2 cups fresh baby spinach
½ cup blueberries, fresh
4 tablespoons lemon juice
1 tablespoon chopped fresh mint

Directions:

In a food blender combine all ingredients.

Process until smooth.

Serve after.

Conclusion

I hope you enjoyed the recipes in this book and that you were successful in eating clean. Remember, you only have one body, so it's good to take care of it.